MODERN TEXTBOOK OF PERSONAL AND COMMUNAL HEALTH FOR NURSES

MODERN TEXTBOOK OF PERSONAL AND COMMUNAL HEALTH FOR NURSES

*Including bacteriology
and the principles of asepsis*

by M. A. PRIEST

*Director of Nurse Education
Bristol School of Nursing
Bristol Health District (Teaching)*

FIFTH EDITION

WILLIAM HEINEMANN
MEDICAL BOOKS LIMITED

LONDON

William Heinemann Medical Books
22, Bedford Square
London WC1B 3HH

ISBN 0 433 26204 4

First published 1960
Second edition 1962; reprinted 1963 and 1964
Third edition, re-set 1966; reprinted 1968 and 1971
Fourth edition 1977
Reprinted 1978, 1983, 1985, 1986

Printed in Great Britain by
Antony Rowe Ltd, Chippenham

CONTENTS

ACKNOWLEDGEMENTS

PERMISSION has kindly been given by Dr Peter Draper and BBC Publications to reproduce Figs 1 and 2 from *The Health Team in Action* (Edited by Bloomfield and Follis). The Controller, H.M. Stationery Office has kindly granted permission for the reproduction of diagrams and tables, including Crown Copyright material, as follows: Figs 3, 11, 12, 13, 14 and 15 from *Management Arrangements for the Reorganised National Health Service*; Fig. 4 from *On the State of Public Health 1973*; the tables on page 98 from *On the State of Public Health 1972 and 1973*; Figs 9 and 10 from *Health and Personal Social Services Statistics for England 1973*; Fig. 16 from *Central Statistical Office 1973*. The original source material for Figs 5, 6, 7, 8 and 17 is also acknowledged to HMSO.

I am grateful to Professor William Gillespie for particular help with the fourth section, and to Dr Geoffrey Tovey for help with the text on the organ matching service. My thanks also to my brother Jack Priest and my friend Miss Diana Eyre-Brook for their generosity and forbearance.

My publishers have continued to be most encouraging and considerate, especially Mr Owen Evans and Miss Ninetta Martyn.

M.A.P.

PREFACE TO THE FIFTH EDITION

MY MAIN task in preparing this fifth edition has been to re-write the first section in order to bring the reader up to date with the provision of health care, by the reorganised National Health Service, which became operational on 1 April 1974.

It was tempting to retain, as historical background, all the material in earlier editions describing the working of the first twenty-six years of the National Health Service, but I have decided not to, except where it is needed to make the present text meaningful.

Many sections have been revised and enlarged. New sections have been added on the following subjects: The Care of the Dying; Pets and Diseases; Renal Dialysis: The National Organ Matching Service; and the Health Education Service.

I have been encouraged by the increasing circulation of my book to Commonwealth and other countries. The World Health Organisation believes that " The enjoyment of the highest attainable standards of health is one of the fundamental rights of every human being without distinction of race, religion, political belief, economic or social condition ". This concept of *complete well being* is well above the level of current demand. If this work helps to further understanding of healthy living and how to achieve it, I shall feel rewarded.

Bristol, January 1977   M.A.P.

ABBREVIATIONS

This glossary may help in the understanding of the reorganised N.H.S.

A.H.A. Area Health Authority. The main operational tier of the reorganised service.

A.H.A. (T) Area Health Authority (Teaching). An A.H.A. in whose area a teaching hospital is situated.

A.M.T. Area Management Team. Formed from the area team officers in a single district area. Equivalent to a District Management Team (D.M.T.).

A.T.O. Area Team of Officers. Comprises an Area Medical Officer (A.M.O.), Area Nursing Officer (A.N.O.), Area Treasurer (A.T.), and an Area Administrator (A.A.).

C.H.C. Community Health Council. To represent the public's interest. The public " watchdog ".

C.H.S.C. Central Health Service Council. Advises the D.H.S.S.

D.M.C. District Medical Committee. Representative of local doctors and dentists in both the hospital and the community services.

D.M.T. District Management Team. Includes a District Nursing Officer (D.N.O.), District Community Physician (D.C.P.), District Treasurer (D.T.), and a District Administrator (D.A.). In addition there are two DMC members representing consultants and general medical practitioners.

F.P.C. Family Practitioners Committee. Replaced the Executive Council.

J.C.C. Joint Consultative Committee. Establishes liaison between the A.H.A.s and the local authorities.

R.H.A. Regional Health Authority. Intermediate tier between the A.H.A.s and the D.H.S.S. Important in long-term planning and major capital investment schemes.

R.T.O. Regional Team of Officers. Comprises a Regional Nursing Officer (R.N.O.), Regional Medical Officer (R.M.O.), Regional Works Officer (R.W.O.), Regional Treasurer (R.T.) and a Regional Administrator (R.A.).

INTRODUCTION

THE IMPORTANCE OF MENTAL, PHYSICAL AND SOCIAL HEALTH TO THE INDIVIDUAL, THE FAMILY, AND THE COMMUNITY

SOUND mental, physical and social well-being are important factors enabling people to live good lives, plan, maintain and care for their families and contribute actively to community living. The health and social services of this country are directed towards the end of providing them. Doctors, health visitors and midwives do everything possible to give pregnant mothers the opportunity of carrying healthy normal babies to full term. They continue their work in hospital or at home to ensure safe delivery.* Their services remain available until mothers have recovered and are able to care for their children unaided.

Being born, travelling safely through the birth canal, is the first hazardous journey in life. Heredity, through the genes, clearly influences the mental and physical state of the newly born child; and if that is satisfactory and if the baby is born safely and starts to breathe lustily a good beginning to life has been made.

The first breaths are vitally important because the brain cells depend on them for their supply of oxygen. Separated from mother, a separate entity for the first time, the infant's brain could be damaged in the first few moments of life if deprived of oxygen.

Subsequent growth and development of body and mind, through experience to maturity, depends largely on mental health.

A mature adult wants to earn a living, make decisions, control appetite and give freely of affection. Only thus can one live happily in society, enjoying existence, carrying adult responsibilities, creating a family, and approaching old age with serenity. But one must start with sound mental health.

Physical health, although important, is certainly second in importance to mental health. It is obvious that an individual born with all special senses, and free from physical handicap and disease, has

* In the U.K. in 1974, 92 per cent of deliveries were carried out in hospital.

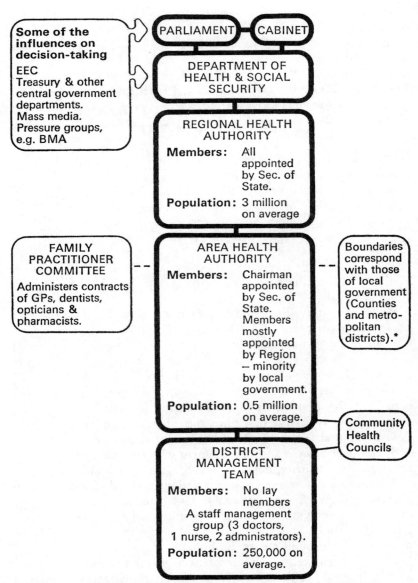

Some of the influences on decision-taking

EEC
Treasury & other central government departments.
Mass media.
Pressure groups, e.g. BMA

PARLIAMENT   **CABINET**

DEPARTMENT OF HEALTH & SOCIAL SECURITY

REGIONAL HEALTH AUTHORITY

Members: All appointed by Sec. of State.

Population: 3 million on average

FAMILY PRACTITIONER COMMITTEE

Administers contracts of GPs, dentists, opticians & pharmacists.

AREA HEALTH AUTHORITY

Members: Chairman appointed by Sec. of State. Members mostly appointed by Region — minority by local government.

Population: 0.5 million on average.

Boundaries correspond with those of local government (Counties and metropolitan districts).*

Community Health Councils

DISTRICT MANAGEMENT TEAM

Members: No lay members
A staff management group (3 doctors, 1 nurse, 2 administrators).

Population: 250,000 on average.

(* Arrangements in Scotland, Wales and Northern Ireland are somewhat different)

See pages 37–40

Fig. 1.   The basic chain of command in the NHS in England* from 1974.

an advantage over someone less favourably endowed. In this present age opportunities are tremendous, but many of the advantages of travel and experience are denied to those with serious physical handicaps.

As a result of preventive medicine and the work of the social services of this country, one sees few cripples under the age of thirty. Crooked backs and legs are rarities. Those born with or having acquired physical handicaps are given every opportunity to pursue some sort of training—training which, in most cases, aims at giving the maximum possible degree of independence. The blind, the deaf and the dumb can all be taught to live useful lives, provided they have a certain degree of mental ability. Dumbness is not a condition in itself; generally it is due to lack of training of the deaf child.

Social stability is as important as physical fitness. There is no rigid line of separation between physical and mental health. Emotional factors working through the central nervous system can produce physical changes in the body causing definite deterioration in health. The changes produce what is called psychosomatic disease. This is a most important condition, for it is stated that 15 per cent of the patients seen by the general practitioner are suffering from psychosomatic illness. It is in this category of disease that the medical social caseworker's help is invaluable.

The science of hygiene is as old as that of medicine. Both have advanced through the ages and made spectacular progress during the last fifty years. Intercommunication and travel have enabled the more advanced nations to share new discoveries and to pass their knowledge to others. Rules founded on common sense are readily accepted throughout the world; to have enough clean food, water and milk; to breathe clean air; to live in dry, clean houses; to dispose of harmful or unsightly waste; to exterminate vermin, mosquitoes, intestinal worms and bacteria; to educate the young; to prevent and cure illness; to provide adequate space for mental, physical and spiritual recreation; to curb excessive habits of drinking, smoking, sex or drug taking.

The phrase " Personal and Communal Health " includes all these aspects. Most countries provide themselves with governments having sufficient authority to create and implement the legislation they need, and such organisations as the World Health are able to offer help to those less well developed.

In the world-wide quest for health there is something for everyone to do. Doctors and nurses have a twofold contribution to make; they seek to restore to health damaged or sick bodies and minds, and are

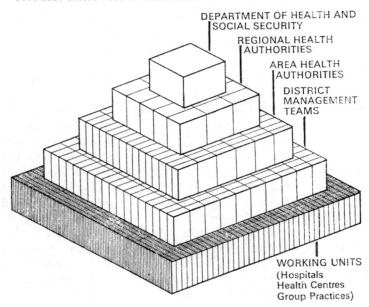

DEPARTMENT OF HEALTH AND
SOCIAL SECURITY

REGIONAL HEALTH
AUTHORITIES

AREA HEALTH
AUTHORITIES

DISTRICT
MANAGEMENT
TEAMS

WORKING UNITS
(Hospitals
Health Centres
Group Practices)

Fig. 2. In England responsibility delegated from central government to working units for the provision
of practically all health care.

very much concerned to teach positive health to all. Teachers, social
workers, parents, in fact all people can contribute in their own
spheres, but the first and perhaps most important step toward that
aim is to keep themselves healthy.

GENERAL SURVEY OF THE HEALTH SERVICE
IN THE UNITED KINGDOM

This is dealt with under two headings:

(1) **Personal Health Services.** These are concerned with the
health of individuals and are available to people normally resident in
Britain according to medical need and without regard to any insurance
contribution. Ministerial responsibility is vested in a Secretary of
State for Social Services in England, and his equivalents in Scotland,
Wales and Northern Ireland. In England, 14 Regional Health
Authorities and 90 Area Health Authorities—16 of them in Greater
London—are responsible, through central government officers, to the
Secretary of State, for the provision of practically all *health* care.
This incorporates *hospital, community and family practitioner* services.*

* See Figs 1, 2 & 3.

REGIONS AND AREAS VARY IN SIZE

Regions	Population of Region	Number of Areas	NUMBER OF AREAS IN POPULATION BRACKETS				
			Under 250,000	250,000 to 500,000	500,000 to 750,000	750,000 to 1,000,000	Over 1,000,000
	(000's)						
Birmingham	5.105	11	1	7	1	1	1
Sheffield	4.283	8	2	1	2	3	—
Manchester	4.107	11	5	4	1	—	1
Leeds	3.501	7	1	3	2	1	—
Newcastle	3.139	9	3	4	2	—	—
South Western	3.024	5	—	3	—	2	—
Wessex	2.518	3	—	1	1	—	1
Liverpool	2.471	6	2	2	1	1	—
Oxford	2.074	6	2	2	1	1	—
East Anglia	1.697	3	—	—	3	—	—
North East Met*	—	1*	—	—	—	—	1
South East Met*	—	2*	—	—	1	—	1
South West Met*	—	2*	—	—	1	1	—
North West Met*	—	2*	—	1	—	1	—
TOTAL		76	16	28	16	11	5

Fig. 3. Regions and areas vary in size.

* Non-London areas only. The four metropolitan regions include London A.H.A.s. These are not included in this analysis.

In Scotland, Wales and Northern Ireland it is considered unnecessary
to have Regional Authorities, thus there is only one administrative
tier (see pages 37–40).

Personal social services including hospital social work and the
home help service, are also controlled by the Secretary of State for
Social Services, but authority for providing social care is vested in
local government. These services are administered at county level by
a Director of Social Services.

(2) **The Environmental Health Services.** The Area Health
Authorities share with local government responsibility for providing a
standard of living environment which is conducive to health and to

VITAL STATISTICS

Age and sex structure of the home population of England at mid-1973

Age (years)	Males (000)	(per cent)	Females (000)	(per cent)	Persons (000)	(per cent)
0–14	5,623.7	24.9	5,332.4	22.4	10,956.1	23.6
15–44	9,153.8	40.5	8,916.7	37.3	18,070.5	38.9
45–64	5,350.1	23.7	5,687.1	23.9	11,037.2	23.8
65 & over	2,453.7	10.9	3,906.8	16.4	6,361.5	13.7
All ages	22,582.3	100.0	23,843.0	100.0	46,425.3	100.0

Age distributions of the population of England: medians[1] and quartiles[2]

	Lower quartile	Median	Upper quartile
1901	11.4	24.0	40.3
1931	15.8	30.4	48.3
1961	16.5	35.8	54.0
1973	16.0	34.2	55.0

[1] The median age divides the population into two equal
halves so that at that time half are younger and half are older.
[2] The quartiles are those ages above (upper) or below (lower)
which lie one quarter of the population of that time.

Fig. 4.

(Reproduced by permission of the Controller of H.M.S.O. from *On the State of Public Health 1973, Annual Report*, pages 11 and 12.

prevention of the spread of disease. In this respect they are therefore concerned jointly in matters of housing, public building and works, transport, water supply, sewerage etc. They are especially involved with regard to the control of infectious disease and health control at sea and airports. This co-operation extends from day-to-day provision of services of mutual concern to the spheres of forward planning and policy making.

PERSONAL HEALTH SERVICES

The National Health Service Act 1946 became operative on 5 July 1948, to provide " A comprehensive medical service designed to secure improvement in the physical and mental health of the people and the prevention, diagnosis and treatment of illness." On 1 April 1974—as the result of further legislation, the 1973 Reorganisation Act—the service underwent complete administrative reorganisation designed to unify the whole structure. The circumstances creating the need for the 1946 Act are interesting historically but within the terms of reference of this book only in summarised form. It was the culmination of a steady improvement in social standards, formulated in the report of the late Lord Beveridge on Social Insurance and Allied Services, published November 1942. The 1973 Reorganisation Act was considered necessary because 25 years of tripartite division into local hospital, local authority and executive council services had failed to achieve an even and fair distribution of health care resources (money and manpower).

During the late nineteenth and early twentieth centuries various Health Acts were administered by local government boards. After the First World War, 1919, their powers were vested in the Ministry of Health and administered through the local authorities. In 1936 an Act to consolidate the remaining advantages of the Public Health Acts of 1848 to 1857 became the guiding light.

The need for Government action to preserve health and manpower gained recognition largely through recruiting experiences in three wars; the Boer War, and the First and Second World Wars. Throughout the period drug and hospital costs tended to rise beyond the reach of average wage-earners and although the expectation of life was constantly rising the standard of health and the loss to the community from sickness and disablement caused much concern. Furthermore medical progress had increasing benefits to offer but could not develop them without ever-increasing fiancial support. The legislative machinery repeatedly got out of date and had to be

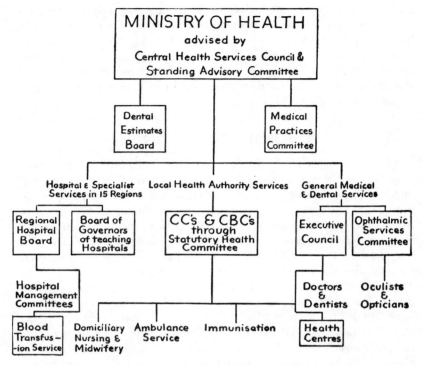

Fig. 5.   The National Health Service Act, 1946.

renewed; and a milestone in that process was the National Health Act 1946 (see Fig. 5).

It changed the pattern of health service administration substantially. It provided *inter alia* for campaigns to promote preventive medicine; the names National Health Service and School Health Service are symptomatic of this intention. Accepting positive health as a communal responsibility, a national aim, a condition enabling each individual to live in harmony with his environment, it challenged the community to raise its general level and stimulated each citizen to rise with it. It was part of a wider pattern of social progress which could not be regarded as entirely separate from others such as the Education Act of 1944, the Factory Acts of 1937 and 1948, and the Children Act 1948.

Even so, by the 1960s criticism suggested that preventive medicine was still not receiving its just share of money and manpower; the emphasis was still toward curative work; and the chronically sick and mentally sick members of the community were by comparison very deprived of money and manpower resources.

On 5 July 1948 all the hospital, specialist, and public health services became the responsibility of a Minister of State. Once appointed with specialist advisers to help him he channelled much of his work through the local authorities but the new concentration of power at government level made possible, for the first time, much coordination between health and community services that could not otherwise have been achieved. Even so, events proved this co-ordination to be insufficient. The dominance of hospital-based attitudes and values throughout the N.H.S. and poor liaison between staff working in the community services and those in the hospitals, resulted in imbalance of standards of care. The fact that the service was divided into three parts, each separately managed and financed, led to the setting up of artificial barriers, which had an adverse effect on the provision of patient care. It was this tripartite administration pattern that has, to a large extent, been blamed for the unfair distribution of resources and manpower.

The Reorganised Health Service

The whole purpose behind reorganisation is to provide an integrated patient-centred service, making full use of all available resources of money and manpower, in an effort to satisfy the community's health needs. These needs are comprehensive and include inpatient, residential and domiciliary care for preventive and promotive health and for curative medicine.

A vital part of reorganisation is the involvement of the doctor in an advisory role in management and administration at each level through statutory medical committees.

The operation units are 90 Area Health Authorities (A.H.A.s) whose boundaries match those of the non-metropolitan counties and the metropolitan districts of local government. For the day-to-day management and running of the service the A.H.A. is responsible through subdivisions of districts which normally have a population of 150,000–300,000. This is thought to be the smallest population for which the full range of general health and social services can be provided. Of the A.H.A.s in England about one-third are " single district " areas; the remainder contain between 2 and 6 districts.

There are 14 Regional Health Authorities (R.H.A.s) in England and these complete the chain of responsibility to the Department of Health and Social Security and the Secretary of State. In regions, areas and districts, multidisciplinary teams of officers are established to support the authorities (see Figs. 7 and 8).

Hospital Services

Between 1948 and 1974 hospitals and specialist services were controlled by boards of governors or management committees, and

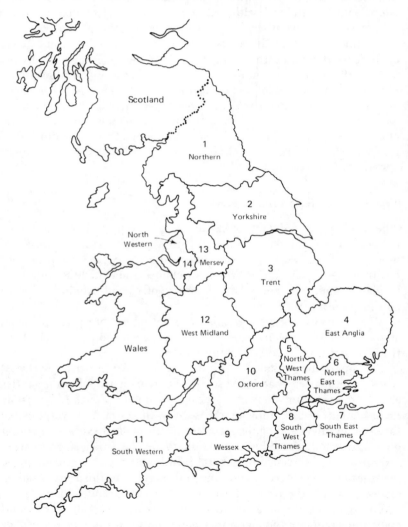

Fig. 6 Map identifying the 14 Regions into which England is divided for the purpose of administering the integrated National Health Service.

DELEGATION FROM THE SECRETARY OF STATE DOWNWARDS
WITH CORRESPONDING ACCOUNTABILITY UPWARDS

FRAMEWORK OF THE ORGANISATION STRUCTURE

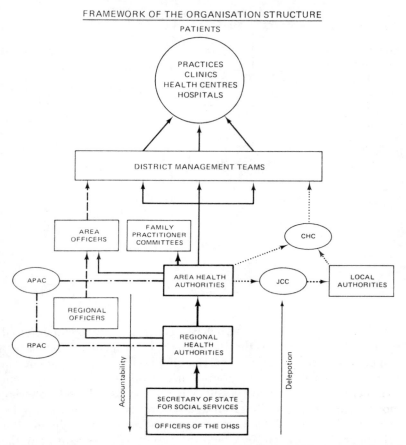

Fig. 7 The whole purpose of reorganisation—to effect the greatest possible decentralisation and delegation from the Secretary of State to the R.H.A.s and from the R.H.A. to the A.H.A.s.

accounted for over half the total cost of the service each year. Hospitals attached to medical faculties of universities were designated " teaching " hospitals and the boards of governors who managed them were responsible directly to the Minister. Other hospitals, excluding a few independent (disclaimed) ones, were controlled by Regional Boards, fifteen of which covered the whole of England and Wales.

Group management committees provided specialist services and made them available for use by local authority health services and by general practitioners. Since 1 April 1974 all hospitals have been

1974 ORGANISATIONAL STRUCTURE, ENGLAND

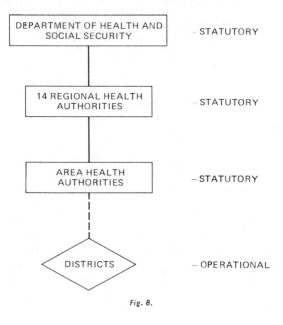

Fig. 8.

grouped into convenient Districts, the control of which is monitored by the Area Health Authority. District Management Teams are responsible for the delivery of Health Service care to patients in hospital as well as in the community. Both in- and out-patient treatment is free but some hospitals have " amenity " beds, offering more privacy than can be given in large wards, for which a supplementary charge is made. Certain hospitals retain the right to offer private accommodation for which the patient is expected to pay the whole cost, together with the cost of other services he receives. This causes controversy and as different governments assume control so the controversy swings for and against the continuation of private beds. Certain amendments have been made since 1948 to reduce the burden of cost falling on the taxpayer. Depending on the government in power a charge may or not be made for each prescription dispensed, and some appliances may have to be partially paid for by the users. Patients unable to afford the charges, however, are given financial assistance through the agency of the social worker.

About 5 per cent of people resident in Britain choose to buy medical care in addition to those who come to this country, especially from the Middle East, for the specialist services we are able to provide.

Excluded from all these provisions are the " Disclaimed " hospitals, most of which were formerly private hospitals.

Community Services

Whereas hospitals and general practitioners are concerned mainly with curative medicine, community services are provided to prevent disease. Between 1948 and 1974 the local authority established a health committee to supervise these services. The person in charge, a medical administrator, was called a Medical Officer of Health, and he was responsible for a wide range of public health services. Health centres; maternity and child welfare clinics; domiciliary midwifery service; health visiting; home nursing; vaccination and immunisation; ambulance service; prevention of disease and after-care; domestic home help and mental health service. The Medical Officer of Health was also designated Principal School Medical Officer. To help him he had a number of senior officers each in charge of a department. As with the hospital services most were free except the Domestic Home Help Service and this was, and still is, subject to a means test.

The Local Authority Social Services Act 1970 caused the Domestic Home Help Service and the Mental Health Service to be transferred to the authority of the Director of Social Services and the reorganisation on 1 April 1974 brought the administration of all the other services into the care of the Area Health Authority. This authority delegates the running of most of the services to the District Management Team, while some of the services are more conveniently organised and supervised at Area level, e.g. School Medical Services.

The term Medical Officer of Health is now obsolete. The medical practitioner dealing with this aspect of the work is called a Community Physician—see reorganised service (Framework of District Organisation Fig. 12 page 21).

General Practitioner Services

Until 1 April 1974 general practitioner services were controlled by 138 executive councils each controlling areas coterminous with those of local authorities in the then counties or county boroughs. They were responsible for dental, pharmaceutical, ophthalmic and domiciliary medical services. They depended on separate advisory committees for the individual services and had available additional resources to meet special needs. It was the executive councils that replaced the National Health Insurance Committees of 1948.

In the unified integrated service the family practitioner services

HEALTH SERVICE STATISTICS

Hospital Summary

	1954	1961	1971	1972
In patients				
Discharges and deaths				
(thousands) *of which*	4,119	4,852	6,207	6,278
private in-patients*	72	84	115	120
Average number of beds				
occupied daily (thousands)	483	457	421	415
of which private in-patients	3	3	3	3
Average length of stay (days)				
All patients	42.8	34.5	24.7	24.2
Excluding psychiatric, geriatric and chronic sick patients	—	14.5	10.4	10.2
Waiting lists (thousands)	—	—	578	563
of which surgical patients	—	—	539	527
Out-patients (excluding accident and emergency)				
New patients (thousands)	—	10,219	10,580	10,435
Average attendances per new patient	—	3.5	4.0	4.1
Accident and emergency patients				
New patients (thousands)	—	5,402	9,054	9,283
Average attendances per new patient	—	2.5	1.7	1.6
Rates per 1,000 population				
In-patients:				
Discharges and deaths	83.4	94.2	114.9	115.7
Waiting lists	—	—	10.7	10.3
Out-patients (excluding accident and emergency):				
New patients	—	199	196	192
Accident and emergency patients:				
New patients	—	105	168	171

* England and Wales only.

Fig. 9.

HEALTH SERVICE STATISTICS

Manpower Summary

	1965	1969	1972
Hospital Services			
Medical staff*	22,123	25,674	29,360
Hospital dental staff*	663	840	938
Hospital nursing staff	264,683	300,598	350,330
Hospital midwifery staff	17,333	19,438	20,680
Hospital professional and technical staff*	31,659	37,930	44,328
Hospital ancillary staff	241,037	257,351	274,189
Hospital administrative and clerical staff*	41,767	48,392	57,140
Regional hospital boards headquarters staff	5,755	7,314	9,736
Mass radiography units and blood transfusion units staff	3,414	3,762	4,042
General Practitioner Services			
General medical practitioners	24,260	24,239	25,184
General dental practitioners	11,572	11,761	12,332
Ophthalmic medical practitioners	887	950	988
Opticians	7,317	6,729	6,639
Executive councils' staff*	4,467	5,266	5,609
Dental estimates board*	1,435	1,387	1,450
Joint pricing committees, drug accounts and pay accounts committee staff*	2,102	2,266	2,146
Local Authority Services			
Nursing staff*	23,854	25,201	28,685

* Whole-time equivalent.

Fig. 10.

are administered by a committee of the Area Health Authority. This is known as the Family Practitioner Committee and provides services for the independent contractors to the National Health Service. Each committee consists of 30 members, half appointed via the local representative committees of the various groups involved, 8 doctors; 3 dentists; 2 pharmacists 1 ophthalmologist; 1 optician; and 15 lay members (non-professional). Of these 15, 4 are appointed by the local authority and 11 by the Area Health Authority.

Under the new service the doctor–patient relationship remains the same. In order to look after patients properly, doctors and dentists have clinical autonomy which enables them to accept full responsibility for the treatment that they prescribe. They therefore remain their own managers, accountable to their patients for the quality of care they give. As in the past they continue to make claims on the resources of the service, but now have more opportunity to be involved in the management of the service.

Individual practitioners are members of Health Care Planning Teams; elected representatives and consultants are members of District Management Teams and some are members of Professional Advisory Committees for re-established Area and Regional Health Authorities.

Services from doctors, since 1948, are free to all normally resident in the United Kingdom according to medical need and without regard to insurance contribution except as modified by amendments to the Act. Only a small minority of the population do not avail themselves of their benefits. People are free to seek doctors of their own choosing and doctors are free to refuse their services. Accepted patients are registered on the accepting doctors' panels. Those requiring medical attention away from home can receive it, the attending being paid from a special fund without loss to the home doctor. These arrangements are specially necessary in seaside areas during holiday periods. The family doctor is the main link between his panel patients and all the health services for them.

It is not mandatory upon doctors to take part in the N.H.S. A few (about 2 per cent) are engaged entirely in private practice. The majority, however, partake in the service full time, while others combine the two.

The average size of the general practitioner's list is between 2,000 and 3,000 patients. A minority of doctors work single-handed practices; the majority partnerships of between 2 and 5 doctors. Many provide antenatal care for expectant mothers and take part in child welfare work. This is done in health clinics and health centres. The growth of primary health care teams has been accelerated since 1972. By the end of 1973, 78 per cent of health visitors and 77 per cent of home nurses were working in association with general practitioners and ancilliary staff.

There are about 25,000 general practitioners in Britain and they are consulted by patients about four times per average patient per year, about 30 times per doctor per day. Doctors and dentists have clinical autonomy; they are therefore their own managers accountable to the patients for the quality of the care they give, but they have claims on the resources of the N.H.S. services. They aim to give continuity of medical care and should receive support from hospitals' diagnostic departments. Doctors are entitled to reasonable working hours and are not under an obligation to obviate all inconvenience to patients and employers. Employers should allow time from work to see the doctor and to assist in the continuity of care. Deputising arrangements are essential. All diagnostic services are based in hospitals for economic reasons, this includes a full range of pathological, radiological and cardiographical services. For economic reasons experience and scarce resources should be used with discretion.

Monetary loans are available to facilitate extending and improving premises and doctors are given every encouragement to make use of shared clinic premises. By 1973 there were 468 health centres established from which about 2,550 family doctors practised, a further 148 were being built and 250 were in various stages of planning.* Middlesbrough has the largest health centre in this country. It houses 21 family doctors serving 60,000 patients. Careful planning allows practices to retain identity while encouraging cooperation with nursing and social service staff. The Central Health Services Council advises the Department of Health and Social Security which provides a health centre design guide. While the health centres provide good facilities and opportunities for teamwork in primary health care, successful working depends on the attitudes and cooperation of those who use them. Medical participation is essential in the management of the service at all levels. An accurate knowledge of current clinical activities largely determines the quality and quantity of calls made upon the service. Users can contribute to the success of the service by using it wisely. By seeking advice when noticing unusual symptoms but not bothering the doctor unnecessarily with minor complaints, and by not expecting an x-ray or a prescription—it may not be necessary. Avoid ill health by eating less if overweight, taking plenty of exercise, limiting or stopping smoking and avoiding excesses of alcohol, or indeed of any kind.

The District Management Team (D.M.T.)

Within each area authority there is a division into districts, which serve as the basic organisation unit for the planning and provision of health care in response to local requirements.

In general, the relationship between the levels of organisation may be seen as a progression from strategic planning and control at the centre to practical activity at the periphery.

---

* By the end of 1975 3,500 general medical practitioners (17%) were practising in health centres, and 634 centres were established with 94 still being built. 146 centres are at planning stage.

DISTRICT ORGANISATION CAN BE REGARDED IN TERMS OF A 3-DIMENSIONAL MODEL

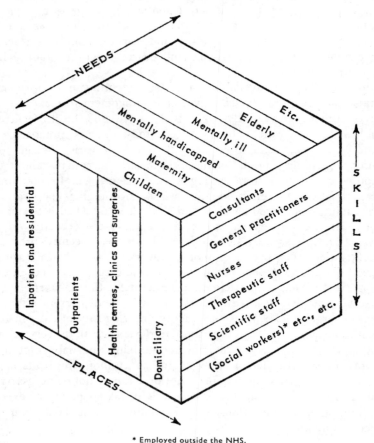

* Employed outside the NHS.

Fig. 11. Management Arrangements for the Reorganised National Health Service.
(By permission of the Controller of H.M.S.O.)

Throughout the structure multi-disciplinary management teams exist to aid the statutorily responsible authorities in the execution of their duties.

It is at the district level that health care is planned and co-ordinated to cater for the specific needs of the local population. By district organisation members of all the health care professions are together involved in evaluating and managing the services they provide.

The districts are seen as the smallest sized units for which substantially the full range of general health and social services can be provided and the largest ones within which all types of professional staff can actively participate effectively in various aspects of the management process through effective representative systems (see Fig. 11).

A typical district in England will have a population of about a quarter of a million. The district boundaries have been defined " naturally "—that is, with primary regard to the population's present use of community and hospital services rather than to the boundaries of the new health area. On the whole, districts are larger and therefore not coterminous with the local authority non-metropolitan county districts through which the environment health services are administered. The same applies to the areas covered by social work teams, each of which usually serves around 50,000 people.

The size of the main health care groups in an average district of 250,000 people is:

About 60,000 children, of whom 500 physically handicapped and 200 severely mentally handicapped.

About 35,000 people over 65, around 4,500 of them severely or appreciably physically handicapped. About 800 would be in hospital at any one time and a similar number in old people's homes, and 1,000 would require domiciliary care.

About 2,000 severely or appreciably physically handicapped people of working age would be living in the community.

About 700 people would be officially classified as severely mentally handicapped of whom over half would be living outside hospitals. At any one time about 300 mentally retarded people would be hospital in-patients.

The total number of people thought as being mentally ill and in contact with hospitals would be around 2,500. Of these, nearly 600 would be in-patients at any one time.

About 19,000 people would need acute medical or surgical care each year as hospital in-patients, about 550 of them being in hospital at any one time.

It is interesting to note that although approximately two-thirds of the N.H.S.'s resources are devoted to providing acute medical care, the needs of the chronically ill and handicapped may be considered to be greater.

The key features of the district organisation include:

(a) District Management Team (D.M.T.s)
(b) District Medical Committees (D.M.C.s)

(c) Health Care Planning Teams. (H.C.P.T.s)

(d) Community Health Councils (C.H.C.s)

Each management team is composed of a nursing and a finance officer, an administrator and a specialist in community medicine (a community physician). It also has two members of the District Medical Committee (D.M.C.)—usually the chairman and vice-chairman who represent consultants and general practitioners. The team is assisted by a number of district officers. (In districts which contain teaching hospitals, representatives from those will also attend and advise the D.M.T. meetings.)

The team as a whole are considered jointly responsible to the appointing A.H.A., which means that in the event of a difference in opinion between team members, the A.H.A. will be called upon to resolve the issue concerned. The four non-elected D.M.T. officers are individually responsible to the A.H.A. as the heads of their respective managerial hierarchies.

The ten members of the District Medical Committees are composed of both hospital and community medical staff (including dentists), so combining many of the functions of the previous hospital medical executive committees with a system of general practitioner representation. The role of the D.M.C. to the D.M.T. is important— it is representative rather than a delegated role. The D.M.T.s make their own decisions but in the light of information made available to them by the D.M.C.

The Health Care Planning Teams conduct detailed local planning to enable the D.M.T. to decide on development of services etc.

The Community Health Councils act as the public " watch-dog " and mouthpiece with regard to the development of the health services.

Health Care Planning Teams

These are multidisciplinary health care planning groups set up within districts by the District Management Teams (D.M.T.s). The composition is adjusted to suit particular situations, but generally will contain general medical practitioners, consultants, nurses, health visitors, relevant paramedical staff and representatives of local authority services particularly social services. The group is supported by the district physicians and an administrator and each team has its own chairman. The chairman has a vital role in securing the good working relationships necessary for cooperation in planning.

There are two forms of Health Care Planning Teams. The first

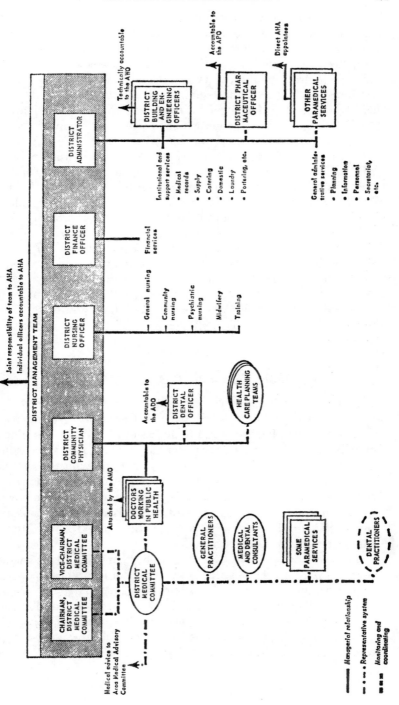

FRAMEWORK OF THE DISTRICT ORGANISATION

are permanent teams with continuous responsibilities and are especially needed where a high level of interaction is necessary between hospital and community care. These services are those with most to gain from integration and unification and involve the elderly, children, maternity services, the mentally ill and the mentally handicapped. National and regional policies guide the D.M.T.s and help to achieve uniformity of these services. The second form of H.C.P.T.s are *ad hoc* groups which disband on completion of the project. Examples of such group activities are the review of primary care services, introduction of day services, reorganisation of out-patients' departments and review of services for people with epilepsy. The aim of H.C.P.T.s is mainly to assess need in order to bring about change resulting in improved standards of care; to identify gaps in relation to needs and to suggest ways of improving services and using existing resources to greater advantage, more economically. They may examine ways of changing existing patterns of care and make proposals to the D.M.T.s which may influence decisions on operational policies, procedure and priorities. Findings of the H.C.P.T.s assist the A.H.A.s and the D.M.T.s develop annual area and district plans. The D.M.T.s may use these groups to monitor and coordinate the implementation of projects and to assess the results.

Community Health Councils (C.H.C.s)

The public, consisting of consumers of health care provided by the N.H.S., makes its voice heard through *Community Health Councils* the membership, functions and resources of which are determined by ministerial regulations. The Secretary of State refers to these councils as " the teeth of publicity ". The Councils provide the means by which the community as a whole exercises its right to express its views about the service. To do this, the Councils have the power to secure information, the right to visit hospitals and other insititutions, and access to the Senior Officers of the Area Health Authority administering the District Services.

The composition of a C.H.C. is important. Half of its members are nominated by the District Council (the local authority), one-third by local voluntary bodies and the remaining one-sixth by the Regional Health Authority. However, provision is made for local variation and experimentation. The total membership is between 20 and 30.

Each Council appoints its own chairman, publishes its own report, communicates to the A.H.A. the views of patients, the needs, priorities and deficiencies of the service. Arrangements are made for the Council to meet A.H.A. officials at least once a year.

The A.H.A. has an obligation to respond by taking appropriate action. It is expected to publish its comments on the Council's findings and the action it has taken or intends to take.

The functions of the Community Health Council must be seen as quite distinct from those of the A.H.A.'s complaints machinery and of the *Health Services Commissioner*. The Council is seen as the public's watchdog whose prime purpose is to represent the community it serves, to establish harmonious relationships with other communal bodies concerned with the promotion of health and to devise means of ascertaining the community's views on the manner in which health care is being provided.

The Council must be consulted by the A.H.A. before decisions are taken on any substantial development or variations in service. The D.M.T. is expected to establish close links with the C.H.C. although there is no formal link.

The central government provides for a *National Council* to advise and assist the C.H.C.s effectively to fulfil their role as the local representatives of users of the health services.

National Council
The Council, which has its own director, provides a national voice. It can arrange conferences for its members and staff of C.H.C.s, can promote and finance research into methods of ascertaining the views of users of the health services and can undertake or arrange surveys of opinion on behalf of A.H.A.s.

Health Services Commissioner
The consumer also has a voice and protection through *A Health Services Commissioner* who works on Ombudsman lines and who will investigate cases which are not satisfactorily dealt with by the appropriate professional body or an ordinary court of law.

Medical Committees

These are formed and function separately at district, area and regional levels. They are formed by a cross-section of representative medical practitioners at all levels of seniority. Members are chosen by hospital, medical or cogwheel executive committees. At each level, they advise their respective authority and team of officers on all matters pertinent to health care.

The Area Health Authority

This is the lowest level of statutory authority and is collectively responsible to the R.H.A. for providing comprehensive health care services to the people of its area. Individual officers may have delegated powers which make them individually accountable for certain services.

Membership of the Authority varies between 15 and 28 people representing those from local government (housing and environment) and health service employees. A chairman is appointed by the Secretary of State and he is supported by a team of four officers (A.T.O.s). These are the only members of the Authority receiving direct payment in addition to expenses. An area which includes a university with a medical faculty or a teaching hospital has additional members and is designated an Area Health Authority (Teaching) (A.H.A.(T.)). In a single district area they act as a District Management Team (D.M.T.).

The A.H.A.s employ most of the N.H.S. staff and have full operational and considerable planning responsibility. The Authority is responsible for assessing needs in its area and for planning, organising, and administering health care services to meet them. D.M.T. proposals for planning and budgeting, based on A.H.A. guidelines, are put to the Authority and after reviewing, and where necessary challenging these proposals, the A.H.A. agrees a budget for each district. The A.H.A. appoints the D.M.T.s other than the elected members.

The A.H.A. has a responsibility to see that their own services and those of the local authority such as social services are organised in a mutually supportive and complementary manner. It may arrange for mutual attachment of staff who can act in advisory or executive roles.

Joint Consultative Committees (J.C.C.s) are set up to discuss and coordinate policies. In London one such committee exists to cover all services, but in the non-metropolitan areas one covers personal social services and school health and another deals with matters concerning environmental health and housing. The roles of the J.C.C.s may vary considerably, but they exist to help the A.H.A.s determine policies and plan comprehensive and balanced health care services in conjunction with local authorities. Even so, the A.H.A.s must work within national and regional policy guidelines and the resources allocated by the R.H.A.s.

The A.H.A.s plan and organise family practitioner services,

EXAMPLE 2 OF THE A.H.A. ORGANISATION
WITH DISTRICTS

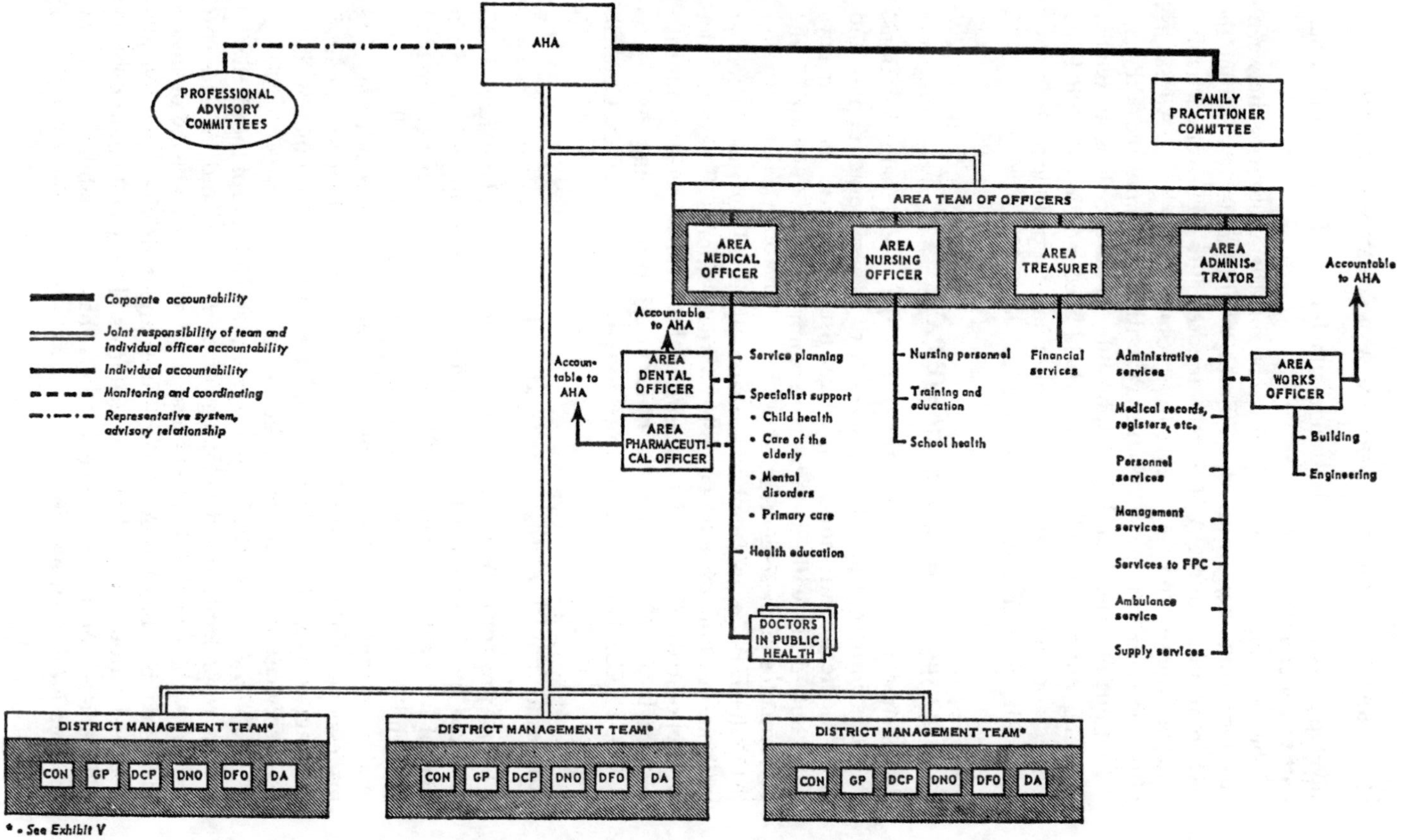

Fig. 13. Framework of the A.H.A. organisation with districts.

AHA

PROFESSIONAL ADVISORY COMMITTEES

FAMILY PRACTITIONER COMMITTEE

AREA TEAM OF OFFICERS

AREA MEDICAL OFFICER
- Service planning
- Specialist support
  - Child health
  - Care of the elderly
  - Mental disorders
  - Primary care
  - Health education

Accountable to AHA

AREA DENTAL OFFICER
AREA PHARMACEUTICAL OFFICER
Accountable to AHA

DOCTORS IN PUBLIC HEALTH

AREA NURSING OFFICER
- Nursing personnel
- Training and education
- School health

AREA TREASURER
- Financial services

AREA ADMINISTRATOR
- Administrative services
- Medical records, registers, etc.
- Personnel services
- Management services
- Services to FPC
- Ambulance service
- Supply services

AREA WORKS OFFICER
- Building
- Engineering
Accountable to AHA

DISTRICT MANAGEMENT TEAM*
CON | GP | DCP | DNO | DFO | DA

DISTRICT MANAGEMENT TEAM*
CON | GP | DCP | DNO | DFO | DA

DISTRICT MANAGEMENT TEAM*
CON | GP | DCP | DNO | DFO | DA

Corporate accountability
Joint responsibility of team and Individual officer accountability
Individual accountability
Monitoring and coordinating
Representative system, advisory relationship

* See Exhibit V

develop health centres and arrange attachment of nurses and other staff to general practices.

The chairman of the A.H.A. acts for the Authority between meetings consulting with the officers where necessary. Although certain members of the A.H.A. take an interest in affairs of particular districts, they do not have executive responsibility. The A.H.A. is responsible for setting up a Family Practitioner Committee (F.P.C.).

In a nutshell the A.H.A. is responsible for all decisions on policy, planning and resource allocation; is held accountable to the R.H.A. for operational control and must monitor and control the performance of its officers at area and district levels.

Family Practitioner Committee (F.P.C.)

Established by the A.H.A., the F.P.C. has four main functions. It enters into contracts for services with general practitioners and other medical contractors; it prepares lists of practitioners; it pays them and deals with disputes and complaints arising out of the performance of these contracts.

Of the F.P.C.s 30 members, 11 are appointed by the A.H.A., at least one of whom must be a member of the Authority. The remainder are appointed by the local authority, the local medical committee and the local committees of the other health professions.

The F.P.C. has replaced the pre-1974 Executive Medical Council.

Regional Health Authorities (R.H.A.s)

The 14 pre-1974 Regional Hospital Boards in England have been replaced by 14 Regional Health Authorities (see map page 9). Such tiers of authority do not exist in Wales, Scotland and Northern Ireland (see end of section). Each Authority has 15 members, all directly appointed by the Secretary of State, and each has a team of 5 professional officers to head the 5 main services. These are medical, nursing, works, administration, and treasury. Their function is to head services, not to act as managers.

The R.H.A. is accountable to the Secretary of State of the D.H.S.S. and is responsible for developing strategic plans and priorities in accord with N.H.S. policies. These are based on a review of needs identified by the A.H.A. and its judgement of the right balance between various areas' claims on resources. The R.H.A. monitors the A.H.A.'s performance and each R.H.A. has responsibility for up to 11 Area Health Authorities.

FRAMEWORK OF THE RHA ORGANISATION

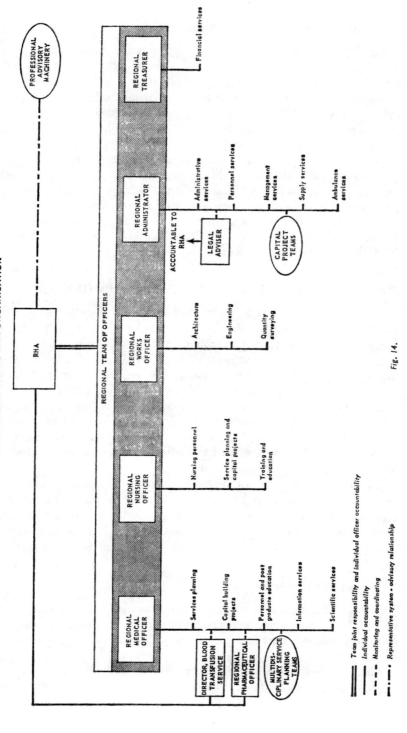

Fig. 14.

The R.H.A. is responsible for identifying, after consulting with its A.H.A.s, services such as blood transfusion, which require a regional approach for providing these services. It is also responsible for managing the design and construction of major building projects as well as providing highly specialised management services such as computing and operational research. It supports and coordinates facilities for teaching and research.

The R.H.A. appoints and arranges contracts for consultants and senior registrars of non-teaching hospitals. It appoints A.H.A. members except for the salaried chairman, who is appointed by the Secretary of State, and the local authority representatives.

The R.H.A. provides the link between the A.H.A.s and the Secretary of State for the D.H.S.S. Members exercise authority only when meeting as members.

The Department of Health and Social Security (D.H.S.S.)

The section of the D.H.S.S. involved in the administration of the Health Service is divided into six functional groups. Each group is composed of professional members with supporting staff. The D.H.S.S. is ultimately responsible for policy decisions affecting the future of the N.H.S., and has a particular role in forecasting future staff requirements and consequent need for training places.

Expert advice is made available to the D.H.S.S. through various advisory bodies, the most important of which is *The Central Health Service Council* (*C.H.S.C.*). A group—*The Personal Social Services Council* (*P.S.S.C.*) has replaced the Advisory Committee on Health & Welfare of Handicapped Persons.

To increase democracy in the N.H.S., the Government is currently looking at membership of Health Authorities and Community Health Councils. The aim is to develop the latter into a powerful forum where consumer views can influence the N.H.S. and where local participation in the running of the N.H.S. can become a reality.

The Cost of the Service

The cost of all these services is understandably heavy and ever rising. It is met from general taxation, 82 per cent; insurance contributions, 8½ per cent; local rates, 6 per cent; and charges 3½ per cent.

Although much has been achieved since 1948 there is room for improvement. More efficient use needs to be made of facilities and

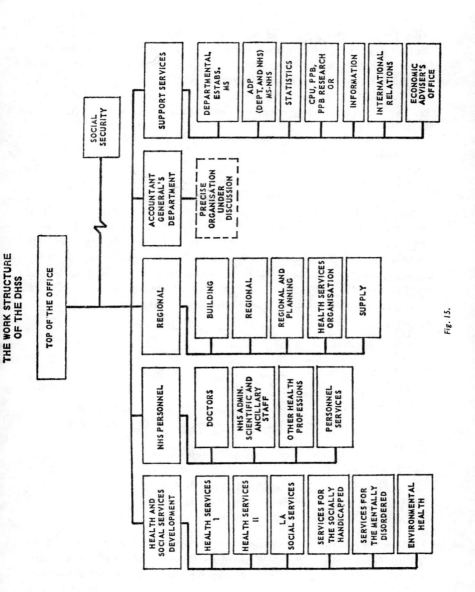

THE WORK STRUCTURE OF THE DHSS

Fig. 15.

staff, better buildings are needed and all forms of waste must be stopped.

In 1972–3, £2,694 million was spent in running the N.H.S. Of this total 58 per cent was for running hospitals, 25 per cent for running general practitioner services, 8 per cent for new building and 3 per cent on other services and administration. By 1974 it was estimated that the total running cost had risen to £5,000 million.

The N.H.S. employs $3\frac{1}{2}$ per cent of the working population and 20 per cent of all people with further education qualifications.

Environmental Health Services

This is the *second* heading of our general survey of the nation's health services (see page 6). The local authorities, besides working under the Department of Health and Social Security in the field of personal health, also work under the Department of the Environment and local government in the field of environmental health. Their efforts in this latter field are directed towards the improvement and maintenance of standards of cleanliness in all aspects of our environment. They work through organisations responsible for implementing the following Acts of Parliament:

(1) Housing and Slum Clearance Acts.
(2) Public Health Act 1936, with reference to
     Sewage and Refuse Disposal.
     Public Nuisances and Offensive Trades.
     Public Water Supplies.
(3) Clean Air Act 1956, concerned with smoke abatement.
(4) Food and Drugs Act 1955, concerned with purity of food and drugs.
(5) Public Health Act 1936 with reference to the prevention of the spread of infection.
(6) Health Services and Public Health Act 1968.
(7) Local Authority Social Services Act 1970.
(8) Health and Safety at Work Act 1974.

The overall purpose of these Acts and of the work of those who enforce them is to provide a healthy environment for all of us so that we may enjoy the full benefit of services provided for us more personally. And although they are not within the scope of this book mention should be made of other fringe benefits, notably the occupational health services provided by industry, which complete the pattern of physical, mental and social welfare that has been created mainly during the last twenty to thirty years.

The Individual as a Citizen. So far we have been concerned with the benefits conferred by the State on the individual. But community welfare has two facets; and the responsibility of the individual to the community should not be disregarded. What does the community expect of the individual citizen?

It expects one to live in a socially acceptable fashion, within the law and in obedience to it; to use its services with consideration and with the restraint demanded by economy; and to commit no nuisance. To have respect for neighbours and consideration for their comfort. To avoid making undue noise or noxious smells. To avoid causing pollution to water supplies or allowing uncleanliness in food. To avoid causing damage to property, public or private, other than one's own. To avoid leaving litter or waste in public places. To prevent the spread of disease and vermin from one's own premises to those of others. And to refrain from assaulting one's fellow men.

The community expects each family to be as far as possible self-supporting, to seek assistance only in real need, and to maintain in its home freedom from disease. To use, but not to abuse, the public services the aim to foster its good health.

The community expects its active adult citizens to protect children, physically handicapped and elderly folk from traffic, fire and flood, physical danger, cruelty and neglect. To use roads for safe travel, to control animals, and to carry the burdens of the community which only they can carry. Part of that burden is the onus of government; of helping to choose it with intelligence and understanding; of supporting it loyally even if he voted with the unsuccessful minority; perhaps of taking an active part in it; and of rearing its future citizens.

The Individual and the Community. Who is the individual and who the community? Clearly the community is the sum of its individuals, but some individuals are greater parts than others. A well-known political philosophy declares that society should expect from each according to ability and give to each according to need. It is a philosophy that in this day and age cuts right across party politics. However they vary in their methods of pursuing it, all parties have become its apostles. Most of us live through stages of giving and taking, and clearly if the community is to thrive there must at any time be as many givers as takers.

PUBLIC EXPENDITURE ON THE HEALTH AND

£ million

	1951–52	1961–62	1972–73	1973–74
Current expenditure				
Hospital, etc., services[2]	275	551	1,885	1,883
less Receipts from patients	−3	−6	−16	−18
General medical, etc., services[2]	166	274	678	735
less Receipts from patients	−4	−41	−74	−80
of which (net cost):				
Pharmaceutical services	53	77	257	283
General dental services	36	52	102	111
General ophthalmic services	10	10	15	16
General medical services	59	88	212	229
Local authority services:				
Health	38	82	173	198
Personal social services[3]	29	56	372	448
School meals and milk:				
School milk[4]	10	14	9	9
School meals	42	85	257	325
less Payments by parents	−16	−35	−102	−111
Welfare foods[2]	32	29	13	12
Departmental administration, other services, etc.	7	19	73	100
Total current expenditure	576	1,028	3,048	3,501

As children we cannot but be takers. We do not ask to be born, and those who bring us into the world owe it to us to give us a good start in life, either within the close limits of home life or through government in the wider world of school, college, professional training and initial employment. After that, as adults, we become the givers. And in old age we must become takers again; for even if we accumulate enough savings to support comfortable retirement our money is worthless without the labour of the givers.

That is of course an over-simplification of a complex concept. Even in adult life, because of differences in natural or financial endowment, some are dependent on others for their opportunities. The adult community must consider its adult members as individuals, accepting a joint responsibility for giving to each an active part to play in life's game. When we consider what the individual expects of the community we must accept that some, because of age,

PERSONAL SOCIAL SERVICES IN BRITAIN[1]

	1951–52	1961–62	1972–73	1973–74
Capital expenditure				
Hospital, etc., services	15	44	231	256
Local authority health and personal social services	7	15	73	105
Other services	6	3	56	16
Total capital expenditure	28	62	310	377
Total public expenditure on health and personal social services	604	1,090	3,358	3,878
Capital and current expenditure (net) expressed as percentage of total expenditure on health and personal social services:				
Hospital, etc., services	47.5	54.0	56.0	54.7
Pharmaceutical services	8.8	7.1	7.7	7.3
General dental services	6.0	4.8	3.0	2.9
General ophthalmic services	1.7	0.9	0.4	0.4
General medical services	9.8	8.1	6.3	5.9
Local authority health services	6.8	8.1	5.7	5.8
Local authority personal social services[4]	5.5	6.0	12.7	13.6

Source: Central Statistical Office.

[1] Including current expenditure on school meals and milk.
[2] Including administration.
[3] Including, from 1969–70, some services transferred from local authority health services.
[4] Expenditure on school milk was borne by the central government in 1951–52.

Fig. 16.

ability, inheritance, position, physical endowment or just pure chance have more responsibility than others for organising society to provide it.

What does the individual expect of the community? A healthy start with enough good food, adequate clothing and a competent home. If the parents cannot provide these things unaided they must become the responsibility of society in general. Protection in childhood from mental, physical and moral danger. Room to grow, learn and play. Love and affection from parents or parent-substitutes. Education, according to the well-known words of the 1944 Education Act, to suit age, ability and aptitude, and to equip one to play a part in the drive for good health. Medical attention, social adjustments and acceptance, and such special training as may be needed to compensate for sub-normal natural endowments. And moral guidance from home, church and school.

Then a place in society as a wage-earner, salaried professional or profit-making trader; a fair deal from employers in return for fair service; a place to live within one's means; a place in a society able to organise the mechanics of its everyday life, with clean food to buy, clean water to use, and adequate refuse disposal.

One expects society to be able to eliminate nuisance from neighbours and travellers, and danger from bandits; to employ policemen to safeguard property and workmen to tend the district; medical attention in sickness or injury; public amenities such as libraries and swimming baths; public security from armed forces, police and fire brigades; legal advice as accuser or accused and justice as the outcome. The individual expects information about the spending of public money to which each has contributed and opportunity for voicing a protest if this money is wasted.

Each adult has a right to help choose the government, which when in office is expected to limit its functions to essentials. He expects the Press to be left free to inform him on matters of national and international import; the broadcasting authorities to be independent of party pressure; and himself to be free to decide whether to go to church and which church to go to, whether to belong to a club, and how to spend his leisure time. Current controversy about membership of trade unions has a bearing on this freedom; perhaps it is pertinent to consider whether trade unionism is a leisure-time or a working-time activity, or whether the two can in fact be so rigidly separated. Each certainly expects leadership in his employment.

He expects society to take action to protect his children from harmful influence, even though such action cannot be taken without danger to the freedoms outlined in the last paragraph; freedom of the Press, the Radio and the Cinema.

And he expects as his powers wane he will be able to retire from active citizenship without poverty but with appreciation for his work and understanding of his limitations.

He certainly expects *a lot*. So much so that only a highly organised society can hope to provide it all. Throughout a thousand years of steady social progress the United Kingdom has become one of the most highly organised societies of the world. Future generations will have to decide whether the process can continue without bringing about the total eclipse of man as an individual.

THE FUTURE OF THE NATIONAL HEALTH SERVICES IN THE UNITED KINGDOM

The 1974 reorganisation was not intended to change the original goals of the 1946 N.H.S. Act, but rather to change the way of its delivery. It has changed and unified the whole health care administrative structure in the hope that more adequate health care will be delivered fairly throughout the whole population. It is obvious that demand far exceeds that level which present resources are able to provide. In the last 25 years the N.H.S. has become one of the largest civilian enterprises employing around 900,000 people and spending over £5,000,000,000 a year. It is obvious also that the original idea behind the 1946 Act, that in time, less services would be needed, is no longer believed. Peoples expectations rise as provision of care becomes more available. It is therefore imperative that we find a way to make the greatest use of the available resources with the aim of giving the most benefit to a maximum number of people. Selective use must be made in the supply of medical care. The recent integration and unification should permit a more flexible and appropriate allocation of resources and effort throughout the health service.

Until time has elapsed sufficient to allow evaluation, it is impossible to forecast results but undoubtedly further change will be necessary within the next few years. Much will depend on changes within the social environment. The two- and three-tier experimental systems of management may be modified. It remains to be seen whether the parts of the environmental, health and social services remaining under local authority control can be made, together with the remainder of the health services to compliment each other effectively, sufficient to overcome the problems of gaps in the service.

It is hoped that the more closely linked authorities will result in more efficient planning and personnel management. Bureaucracy and local autonomy have to be balanced before the fundamental goal of a fair deal for everyone is met.

The Health Education Service (see Fig. 17)

The Department of Health and Social Security has an important

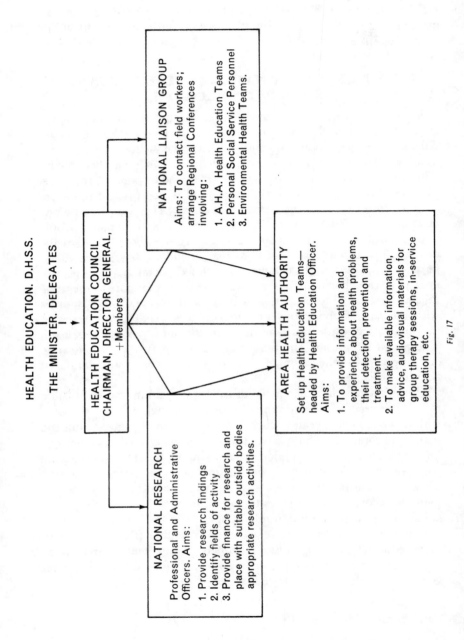

HEALTH EDUCATION. D.H.S.S.

THE MINISTER. DELEGATES

HEALTH EDUCATION COUNCIL
CHAIRMAN, DIRECTOR GENERAL,
+Members

NATIONAL LIAISON GROUP

Aims: To contact field workers;
arrange Regional Conferences
involving:

1. A.H.A. Health Education Teams
2. Personal Social Service Personnel
3. Environmental Health Teams.

NATIONAL RESEARCH

Professional and Administrative
Officers. Aims:

1. Provide research findings
2. Identify fields of activity
3. Provide finance for research and
place with suitable outside bodies
appropriate research activities.

AREA HEALTH AUTHORITY

Set up Health Education Teams—
headed by Health Education Officer.
Aims:

1. To provide information and
experience about health problems,
their detection, prevention and
treatment.
2. To make available information,
advice, audiovisual materials for
group therapy sessions, in-service
education, etc.

Fig. 17

role in promoting health education as a vital part of preventive medicine. The Secretary of State delegates his national responsibility to a Health Education Council. The Council in turn delegates operational responsibility to the Area Health Authorities. To decide on the nature of campaigns and enable the Council to advise the area teams, a research committee, serviced by professional and administrative officers, meets regularly. This committee reviews research findings, identifies fields of activity and makes recommendations regarding the financing of appropriate research. Decisions must also be made as to which are the most suitable agencies to undertake particular research projects.

This committee, in conjunction with the Health Education Council organises and conducts mass-media campaigns, such as those directed against smoking and advocating the need for family planning.

The area teams are directed by a health education officer who has the assistance of other professional workers. Technical and secretarial staff are also employed to give support. The teams make themselves available to the community and are able to supply a wide range of materials for the purpose of influencing opinion. Group therapy sessions can provide a valuable contribution to their work. They also organise in-service education and training sessions for National Health Service staff working in primary and secondary schools.

Arrangements for Reorganised NHS service in Scotland, Wales and Northern Ireland

Scotland with a population of 5.2 million is divided into 15 areas, each with its own Health Board. Responsibility for the central administration of the health services rests with the Secretary of

SCOTTISH HOME AND HEALTH DEPARTMENT

Secretary of State for Scotland
|
He is advised by:
|
1. Common Services Agency
2. Scottish Health Services Planning Council

15 Area Health Boards responsible for setting up suitable management arrangements for themselves

Number of Districts provide the health care needs for the population of 5.2 millions

THE WELSH OFFICE
|
The Secretary of State for Wales
|
He is advised by The Welsh Health Services Technical Organisation
(WHSTO) which carries out a central organisational role, and
The Welsh Council
|

| 8 Area Health Authorities |
| The boundaries are coterminous with the new counties. |
| Provide the health care needs for a population of 2.7 million |

State for Scotland and the Scottish Home and Health Department.
They and the Area Health Boards are helped by two new
bodies: the Scottish Health Service Planning Council and the
Common Services Agency.

The Health Boards are responsible for setting up suitable management arrangements for themselves and deciding on the number of
districts they need.

There is no Family Practitioner Committee structure as in England.
It is the Health Boards that contract for the services and arrange the
payment for medical practitioners, general practitioners, dentists,
pharmacists and opticians.

There is liaison between health and local authority services and
local authority districts with regard to most environmental services
and housing. It is regional liaison with regard to education and social
services. Local Health Councils have similar functioning to Community Health Councils.

Wales with a population of 2.7 million is a health region administered separately from England. In place of a Regional Authority it is
controlled by the Secretary of State for Wales through the Welsh
Office. It is this office that is responsible for the central organisation,
and policy decisions are made on the advice given by a body called
the Welsh Health Services Technical Organisation (W.H.S.T.O.).

The central organisational role is in relation to the eight Welsh
Area Health Authorities, the bounderies of which are coterminous
with the newly formed counties.

Advice on health matters is also given to the Secretary of State
by the Welsh Council.

Collaboration with local authorities is achieved through Joint
Consultative Councils (J.C.C.).

Northern Ireland with a population of 1.6 million reorganised its
health and social service administration six months earlier than
England—in October 1973. Control is by four Health and Social

Service Boards covering different areas. The overall planning is centralised in the Department of Health and Social Security. Help and advice is given by a Central Services Council. A big difference is, that there is one administration; the responsibility for personal social services has been joined with that for health. As in Scotland, medical practitioners, dentists, pharmacists, opticians etc. are in contract directly with the Health and Social Service Boards. The four areas are divided into 26 districts, the boundaries of which are conterminous with the new local government districts. Each district has around 50–100,000 population.

NORTHERN IRELAND
|
Department of Health and Social Security
|
Secretary of State for Northern Ireland
|
He is advised by Central Health Services Council
|

4 Area Health and Social Service Boards. A consortium of which forms the Central Services Agency. This handles matters of common interest centrally. The Area Health Boards have executive authority over the Districts

26 Districts each with its own executive team is responsible for administrating the delivery provision of health care to 1.6 million people

BY COMPARISON:
SUMMARY OF REORGANISED SERVICE IN ENGLAND

ENGLAND
|
Department of Health and Social Security
|
Secretary of State for Social Services
|
Advised by the Central Health Services Council (CHSC) and The Personal Social Services Council (PSSC)
|

14 Regional Health Authorities. Regional Planning. Monitoring the Area Health Authorities within guidelines laid down by D.H.H.S.

90 Area Health Authorities. These are the lowest level of Statutory Authority. They monitor the work of the District Management Team but do not have executive authority over them

Districts provide health care needs to a population of 46.5 million

A consortium of the boards forms a Central Services Agency. Each district has an executive team (D.E.T.) which corresponds to the English District Management Team (D.M.T.) but, unlike the English pattern, the Northern Ireland Area Health and Social Service executive teams have direct authority over the District Executive Teams.

Programme planning teams at area level in Northern Ireland correspond to district health care planning teams in England. District Committees in Northern Ireland correspond to the English Community Health Councils.

PERSONAL HEALTH

PERSONAL hygiene, or rather personal health as we are now tending to call it, is of the utmost importance. So often this subject is thought of mainly in relation to cleanliness of the body, but so many other factors are involved. Cleanliness is important, but also there are other factors equally important if not more so in maintaining the health of the individual. Positive health is something more than cleanliness and absence of disease. It is a state of well-being of the whole body which will enable it to grow and develop normally to its full capacity, and have the ability to enjoy all the opportunities that life may present.

Enough good food*, cleanly prepared and properly cooked, in the right proportions, will provide what is necessary for energy, growth and maintenance. Good posture, exercise and recreation are good for the growing and grown mind and body. Enough rest and sleep and avoidance of fatigue is essential. Good habit formation is valuable, and this can also be applied to the general cleanliness of the body, understanding of the right type of clothing and suitable footwear.

The welfare state, of which we in the United Kingdom have to-day grown so proud, has its dangers. Chief among these can be counted the growth of a generation which tends passively to accept the benefits of sanitary reform, without accepting any personal responsibility for the attainment of positive good health. Too much is taken for granted. This attitude of mind can best be combated by a scheme of health education which lays emphasis on the following main points:

(*a*) The importance of the formation of good habits at an early age, so that these will persist through life—far better than any attempt to get rid of bad habits.

(*b*) The dependence of the health of the community on the sense of responsibility of each individual for his or her own personal health.

(*c*) The probable relationship between the prevalence of certain diseases, deformities and defects, and a faulty way of life.

NUTRITION AND ITS RELATION TO HEALTH

Upon proper nutrition the growth and health of the body are dependent. Nutrition is the process by which food is used by the

* " Recommended Intakes of Nutrients for the United Kingdom " provides an up-to-date and authoritive reference book.

body to produce energy and heat, maintain body function, repair and maintain body structure and promote growth.

The term " A well-nourished child " is often used. By this is meant that the child looks well fed, the food he is getting is suitable and being used to advantage. It is sometimes difficult to decide on appearance and size if a child is well fed, children differ so much in size and general physique, but it is probably true that if a child is healthy he is well fed. By healthy, one means well grown, reasonably well covered, with glossy hair, a good colour, elastic skin and bright alert eyes. He should hold himself well and be alert and enthusiastic.

There is a direct relationship between nutrition and health, and if a child is not healthy various factors require to be investigated. In the first instance, it may be that he is suffering from malnutrition, and there are many reasons for this, the most obvious one being simple lack of quantity of food—not sufficient calories to provide for growth and development. This rarely happens in this country nowadays, but may occasionally occur as the result of poverty and neglect. More often the *quantity* of food is adequate but the *quality* and proportion are at fault. In other words, the child is getting a poorly balanced diet—perhaps sufficient to supply calorie requirements for heat and energy, but not sufficient protein and vitamins. This fault is most often due to ignorance or laziness, and to some extent poverty. The carbohydrate foods are cheaper and on the whole easy to prepare. On the other hand the reason may be quite different; the child may have access to plenty of good food, but because of lack of appetite, which may be due to disease or emotional factors, he will not eat the food provided. Again, he may eat enough food but because of some disease it is not properly digested and utilised. A healthy energetic happy child should enjoy his food and show a steady gain in weight and growth.

So far, nutrition has been emphasised in relation to child health. Not only is it vitally important with children, it is equally important with people of all ages, particularly pregnant women. Our bodies are like complicated machines, which work well provided they are supplied with the proper fuel, and provided the parts are in good working order. If anything interferes with the normal workings of our various systems the nutrition of our body will suffer. For instance, if part of the digestive tract is blocked, by stricture or spasm, the food may be held back and will not get through to the part which deals with digestion and absorption. If on the other hand, there is diarrhœa—aptly described as " intestinal hurry "— then the food will pass through so quickly there will not be time for proper digestion and absorption. If digestive juices are lacking, possibly due to a disease of a particular organ—stomach, intestine, pancreas, liver—or to lack of appetite, then food, if eaten, will not be properly digested and so absorbed. Fever, shock, and emotional disturbances may temporarily interfere with the flow of juices. One knows only too well the feeling of a dry mouth and tongue when one is very nervous. This dry state is reflected further down the tract, and it is often said that the mouth is like a mirror— it reflects the state of the stomach. It is not wise to insist on a patient eating food which requires digestion if, as a result of a high temperature, there is no appetite and consequently a lack of digestive juices. It must not, however, be thought that a patient with a high temperature does not need feeding. The energy used by the body in creating a temperature and fighting an infection needs to be replaced and feeding forms an essential part of nursing treatment. Particularly in long-standing cases of fever sufficient calories must be given but in a form which is easily digestible and quickly absorbed. Glucose, milk and eggs provide valuable amounts of such nutriment. The state of the teeth should also be considered. In children, decayed and broken teeth will interfere with mastication. With adults and elderly people it may be that teeth are absent or dentures are uncomfortable, so that again food is not properly masticated.

Other factors of importance in relation to nutrition and health are sufficient sleep, fresh air and exercise. These, combined with emotional stability, all help to maintain a good appetite and a happy healthy individual.

FOOD AND THE MEASUREMENT OF CALORIES

Food contains the following nutrients which are necessary in various proportions to nourish the body: proteins, fats and carbohydrates. As well as these nutrients, mineral salts, vitamins, roughage and water are essential.

Protein is an essential constituent of all animal and vegetable cells. It is the only nitrogenous food, and consists of the elements carbon, hydrogen, oxygen, phosphorus and *nitrogen*. Protein is used in the body for the growth and repair of tissue, therefore it is particularly important for the growing child, the adolescent, the pregnant mother and the individual having to repair and replace damaged cells, e.g. the badly burnt patient. The word *Calorie* which will occur frequently in the text, means the amount of heat required to raise one kilogramme of water from 0° Centigrade to 1° Centigrade. This is the *large Calorie* and the one used in calculating the heat value of food. The *small calorie* is the amount of heat required to raise one gramme of water one degree centigrade. It is used only on scientific investigations of minute changes of temperature and is one-thousandth part of a large Calorie.

Protein can be used as a source of energy. When eaten, it is acted upon by certain enzymes (digestive fluids) in the stomach and intestine and broken down into amino-acids. There are probably about twenty-six different amino-acids of which about ten are essential for growth. These amino-acids must be supplied by the intake of food and cannot be made by the body. Any one animal protein molecule contains all the essential amino-acids, and so they are spoken of as *first-class proteins*. The first-class proteins are contained in the more expensive foods, e.g. lean meat, fish, eggs, milk and cheese. If food is in short supply these should be well distributed over the day's meals, combined with adequate amounts of fat and carbohydrates. *Second-class proteins* will contain all the essential amino-acids, but not in the right proportions, and not all the essential ones in each molecule, so that a larger quantity is needed to give an adequate supply. Second-class proteins are contained in bread, oatmeal, peas, beans, nuts, wheat, barley, oats, maize and rice, etc. They add roughage to the food and so are of great value. Protein stimulates combustion, it acts rather like a draught on a fire and makes the fire burn more quickly and so increases the output of energy.

First- and second-class proteins eaten in excess of the bodily needs after conversion to amino-acids, are absorbed in the liver. In the liver the nitrogen is extracted and the remaining elements are converted into carbohydrate, to be used as fuel or stored by the body, for reserve use. One gramme of protein yields 4·1 Calories of heat, and about 100 grammes of protein are needed each day for the average adult and children of twelve years or over.

Fats. Fats, like proteins, are derived from two sources, animal and vegetable. They consist of carbon, hydrogen and oxygen and when eaten are digested by enzymes and broken down into fatty acids and glycerine. As such, they are absorbed by the villi of the small intestine into the lacteals and distributed round the body by the lymphatic and blood circulation. In the tissue, fatty acids may be used as fuel or reconverted into fat and stored in the various fat deposits of the body. The fat depots serve to support internal organs, keep them in position, and provide reserve supplies of heat and energy. Too much fat in these depots may prove a disadvantage. Animal fats are probably more valuable than vegetable because they are more easily digested and contain vitamins A and D. For the complete oxidation of fats it is necessary to have suitable proportions of carbohydrate being oxidised at the same time. If this proportion is not correct, fats will be incompletely oxidised and harmful ketone bodies produced. It is these ketones which cause acidosis which is responsible for the coma which occurs in diabetic patients.

One gramme of fat yields 9.3 Calories—100 grammes of fat are required in the diet each day. Animal fats are found in butter, cream, the fat part of any meat, egg yolk and the oils from certain fish. Vegetable fats are obtained mainly from nuts.

Carbohydrates. Carbohydrates are our immediate source of energy for muscular exercise. A carbohydrate molecule consists of carbon, hydrogen and oxygen, and may be in the form of starch or sugar. By means of a complicated and interesting process called photosynthesis, plants are capable of making starch and sugar. In the body these foods are digested by enzymes and converted to simple sugars. As such they are absorbed through the villi of the small intestine and conveyed by the portal system to the liver, where they may be distributed to the tissues for immediate use or converted into glycogen, a form of sugar which can be stored in the liver and muscles. When the body needs an emergency supply of energy, this glycogen can be quickly reconverted and distributed for fuel purposes. Two hormones—adrenaline and insulin—are necessary for this conversion and reconversion. Carbohydrate foods, taken in excess of the body needs, will be converted by the body into fat and stored as such. Foods containing a high percentage of starch are bread, potatoes, all cereals, peas, beans and lentils, and all sorts of flour made from grain. Sugars are obtained from cane or beet sugar and milk lactose. These substances need digesting. Honey and glucose are simple sugars and need no digesting. Cellulose, which is the woody part of stalks of vegetable leaves and fruits, contains carbohydrate, but it is not digested and absorbed. It is, however, valuable in that it provides bulk for the intestine and as such stimulates peristaltic action.

One gramme of carbohydrate yields 4.1 Calories of heat—500 grammes are needed in the diet each day.

Minerals. Unlike protein, carbohydrate and fat, minerals are not taken into account when calculating the energy value of a diet.

Relatively small amounts are required to replace those lost daily through the excretory organs, but they are vitally important, so much so that death may result if they are withheld. Growing children and pregnant women need rather more to allow for growth as well as replacement. There are at least fourteen mineral substances found in the body, most of which are widely distributed in nature and an ordinary well-proportioned diet should provide all that are necessary.

The important functions of these minerals may be summarised as:

(1) To maintain the proper chemical composition of the blood, which preserves the correct reaction and regulates osmotic pressure.

(2) To supply the needs of the growing cells of the body, particularly bones, teeth and nervous tissues.

(3) To act as vital components of many of the body fluids.

(1) *Calcium.*—This is found in milk, cheese and eggs, and in the type of fish which has a bony spine. There is also a little in white bread. Hard water, if not boiled, will supply a reasonable amount; it is good to boil vegetables in hard water, as a quantity of calcium will be precipitated on the vegetables. Calcium is necessary for the growth and maintenance of bones and teeth, the clotting of blood and muscle function. Adequate amounts are especially required during the period of growth, by children and pregnant women. Insufficiency in the diet is to some extent rectified by the parathyroid glands, the secretion of which can divert calcium from the bones to where it is required. Calcium deficiency produces rickets in child and adult, i.e. faulty bones and teeth, failure of the blood to clot and interference with the proper function of body cells. A supply of vitamin D is necessary for the absorption and utilisation of calcium.

(2) *Phosphorus.*—This is well distributed in all animal and vegetable foods, but is not always available to the body. It is usual to assume that if calcium in the diet is adequate, phosphorus will be adequate also. It is essential for healthy bones, teeth and tissue structure, particularly during the period of growth. The adult body can make demands on its stores if it is in short supply in the diet.

(3) *Potassium* is well distributed in all animal and vegetable foods. A balance between calcium, potassium and sodium is necessary for the proper functioning of striped and unstriped muscle and nervous tissue. Potassium is a necessary constituent of body cells and fluids. The amount, and its use in the body, is controlled by the suprarenal cortex and insulin.

(4) *Sodium* is provided by common table salt and milk, bacon, cheese, ham and smoked fish. Loss from the body is to some extent controlled by the suprarenal cortex. Loss may be excessive during intense sweating. It is necessary for all body fluids. Loss of it results in muscular weakness and cramp.

(5) *Chloride* is also provided by common table salt. It is necessary for the manufacture of the hydrochloric acid used in gastric juice and for the maintenance of osmotic pressure. Chloride is not likely to be deficient, since in the event of illness, when the intake is below the body needs, it holds on to its supply and very little will be excreted.

(6) *Iron.*—This is found in very few foods, and on the whole these foods are expensive. It is found in liver, kidney, heart and red meats, sprats, figs, raisins and black treacle. It is essential for the hæmoglobin in the red blood corpuscles, and is also found in the spleen and red bone marrow. Females, particularly during pregnancy, need adequate amounts. Lack of it causes anæmia.

(7) *Iodine* is found in sea fish, particularly herrings, cod and salmon. It is also found in edible seaweeds and in vegetables grown in certain soils, particularly those by the sea. It is contained naturally in some types of water. In this country, and many others, it is added to the drinking water and to the table salt when the water supply is found to be deficient in this element. Iodine is necessary for the manufacture of thyroxin, which is made by the thyroid gland and which controls the rate of metabolism. Only minute quantities are required, but lack of it will cause faulty thyroid function and simple goitre.

(8) *Sulphur* is contained in eggs, milk, meat and cereals. It is needed for healthy hair, nails and body proteins. A mixed diet is not likely to be lacking in it.

(9) *Magnesium* is present in most foods, and is necessary for healthy bones and teeth. Only minute quantities are required, but lack of it will cause serious illness.

(10) *Fluorine.*—Again, only a small quantity is required. It is obtained mainly from drinking water. It has recently become prominent in text books because of the belief that it has a strong influence on the health of teeth. Where fluorine is found to be deficient it can be added to the drinking water. It is said that when added in excessive quantities to drinking water it tends to discolour growing teeth and objections have been raised on this account to adding of fluoride to the local supply. However, in June 1963, the

Minister gave general approval to all local health authorities to the making of arrangements with water undertakers for the addition of fluoride to water supplies which are deficient in it naturally to the level appropriate for the prevention of dental decay.

Other elements are present in small traces in the body, some of which are copper, cobalt, zinc and manganese. None of them are likely to be short in a mixed diet. Cobalt is interesting for its connection with vitamin B 12, and pernicious anæmia; and both copper and cobalt are concerned with the manufacture of blood.

Vitamins. Vitamins have been discovered during this past century, and were first described as " accessory food factors ". Like minerals they are not taken into account when the energy value of food is assessed, but are most important constituents of the diet. Briefly, they can be said to be responsible for the regulation of growth, function and reproduction and only very small quantities are required to maintain good health. Because certain diseases occur through lack of vitamins they are referred to as deficiency diseases. Some vitamins are present in plant life, but others are manufactured as the result of animal cell activity. Vitamins were first referred to by letters of the alphabet, and in many cases they still are, but most of them now have an official name derived from their physiological property or chemical structure.

Vitamins are divided into two main groups—fat soluble and water soluble. Many vitamins can be produced synthetically. Unfortunately, some vitamins are unstable and can be destroyed by heat or alkaline reaction. Vegetables and fruit preserved by cold storage retain their vitamin content.

Deficiency diseases such as scurvy, rickets, beri-beri and pellagra have been known for many years, but it was not until 1912 that the function of vitamins as actual accessory food factors was discovered. Their first name was Vitamine, but since then the " e " on the end has been dropped. Letters of the alphabet were used to identify the different factors, but it is now known that they are much more complex than at first thought. This applies particularly to Vitamin B. Vitamins A, D, E, K are fat soluble. Vitamins B, C are water soluble.

Vitamin A.—This is found in animal fats. In vegetables a substance (carotin) is present which is converted by the body into vitamin A. Sources generally are egg yolk, milk, butter, cheese, fish fats and all yellow vegetables and fruits and green leaves. Vitamin A is necessary for maintaining healthy epithelial tissues capable of resisting infection. It is also necessary for good night vision in dim light, and in some way is responsible for regulating the growth of bone cells. Lack of Vitamin A gives rise to poor night vision and unhealthy epithelial tissues which are less than normally capable of resisting infection. Vitamin A is destroyed by prolonged cooking, and possibly to some extent by dehydration processes. Tinned and frozen foods retain Vitamin A for a limited period. It is known that liquid paraffin interferes with its absorption.

Vitamin D.—Many forms of this are recognised, but two are important, D_2 known as calciferol and made from the ultra-violet ray irradiation of a substance known as ergosterol in the skin; D_3 also occurs in fish oil. It is fortunate that shortage is not a problem in hot climates, where sunshine is abundant. It will only occur if children are confined in dark enclosed homes. Vitamin D is generally found in eggs, butter, cheese, milk and fish fat. It is put by the manufacturers into certain kinds of margarine to fortify them. Provided there is a sufficiency of available calcium and phosphorus, Vitamin D enables bone to calcify normally. It is also necessary for healthy teeth and proper growth of the body. Deficiency may cause rickets in children and osteomalacia in adults. Liquid paraffin hinders the absorption of Vitamin D. Both D_2 and D_3 are known to be equally effective, both can now be manufactured and both are reasonably heat resistant. An excess is more dangerous than a deficit. It increases the absorption of calcium to such an extent that it becomes deposited in the kidneys and elsewhere with disastrous results.

Vitamin E has an official name: Tocopherol. An anti-sterility factor, it is found in wheat germ, egg yolk, milk, green vegetables, especially lettuce. If there is a sufficiency of A, B, C, D vitamins, then E is not likely to be lacking and it is generally believed that the human race does not as a rule suffer from any lack. Its function is not entirely understood. Some authorities believe it to be associated with fertility and to exert some control over it. It is suggested that bile is necessary for its proper absorption and that liquid paraffin hinders absorption.

Vitamin K (anti-haemorrhagic factor)—This vitamin was not considered of any practical importance until about 1939. It is found in foods containing vitamins A, D and C, especially in green vegetables. It is also known to be manufactured by harmless bacteria in the large intestine. Vitamin K is needed for maintaining the prothrombin level in the blood which is necessary for proper clotting. Deficiency is more likely to be due to faulty absorption than to lack of it in the diet. It is not absorbed in jaundice when bile salts are absent in the intestine, or when the absorption of fat is deficient, as in sprue or long standing diarrhoea as in ulcerative colitis. Liquid paraffin also hinders absorption. During long courses of sulphonamides and some antibiotics there may be a deficiency because the intestinal bacteria are, in these cases, greatly reduced. If the mother's diet has been deficient or her absorption faulty, a newborn baby may suffer lack of this vitamin and be subject to hæmorrhagic disease. Extra amounts of vitamin K are necessary for jaundiced patients, particularly if they have to undergo any form of surgery.

Vitamin B.—Water soluble—about twelve different varieties are now described. The functions of all are not understood, but all are fairly widely distributed. All except Vitamin B_{12} are found in bread, meat—especially pork—liver, yeast, oatmeal, green peas, eggs, milk, fruits and potatoes. Most are thought to be destroyed by moist heat, slow cooking and alkaline solutions. Vitamin B complex is subdivided into:

B_1 Aneurin or Thiamin, found particularly in husks of oatmeal and rice. It is necessary for the proper growth and energy output from carbohydrate metabolism. Deficiency causes beri-beri. Intake can be increased during pregnancy and lactation by taking Marmite, Bemax and other B_1 preparations. One of the problems facing millers at the moment is how to produce a white flour without destroying this valuable source of Vitamin B_1.

B_2 Riboflavin is found particularly in yeast, liver, milk and egg yolk. This vitamin is concerned with the normal growth of body tissues and lack of it will cause mucous membrane, skin and eye changes—particularly angular stomatitis (Ariboflavinosis).

B_5 Nicotinic Acid—this is found in yeast and whole cereals. It is essential for carbohydrate and protein metabolism. Lack of it will cause pellagra. The three main symptoms are dermatitis, diarrhœa and finally dementia.

B_4 Biotin—found in liver, kidney, eggs and milk, and in all vegetables. It is not likely to be lacking in a normal diet, but lack of it affects the normal secretions of skin. Thought to be connected with fat and carbohydrate metabolism.

B_6 Pyridoxine is found in liver, fish, egg yolk, yeast and cereals. It was thought necessary for the healthy growth of skin, and proved so on experimental animals, but there is no evidence that it is so in human beings.

Folic Acid—found in yeast, liver and kidney. It affects the manufacture of red blood cells in the bone marrow. It was formerly used in the treatment of macrocytic anæmias.

Cyanocobalamine, or Vitamin B_{12}, is the anti-anæmia substance found in liver and is the extrinsic factor of Castle. It has taken the place of Folic Acid. It is effective in very small amounts in combating pernicious anæmia and preventing degeneration of the nervous system. Liver and kidney are most richly supplied with it, but a little of it is also found in meat, egg yolk and cheese; it can be synthesised biochemically. Patients with sprue may be unable to absorb this vitamin from the gut and so may develop macrocytic anæmia. Other members of the vitamin B group are choline, pantothenic acid, inositol and para-amino-benzoic-acid. Little is known of their value to man at present.

Vitamin C, or ascorbic acid, is found in all fresh fruits, particularly citrus, in fresh vegetables, rosehip syrup and milk. It can be destroyed by faulty cooking but is preserved by plunging the vegetables straight into boiling water and cooking for a short period. Canning and dehydration and freezing do not necessarily destroy it and opinions vary as to whether it is destroyed by the addition of bicarbonate of soda. Vitamin C is necessary for the proper healing of tissue. It is necessary for the building up of the tissue cells, and intracellular substances. Lack of it will cause scurvy, a disease in which growth is slowed down, the mouth and gums become sore, hæmorrhages occur into the tissues and damaged tissue is slow to heal. This applies to both epithelial tissues and bone. People on an ordinary diet should not suffer lack, but those with severe illness appear to need more, particularly if there is extensive damage to tissue.

Vitamin P is found in citrus fruits. It was thought that this vitamin was concerned with normal capillary resistance, but recent publications suggest there is not sufficient proof for this.

Vitamins are usually measured in milligrams or International Units. Deficiencies are rarely single but usually multiple. A mixed diet containing dairy foods, fresh fruit and vegetables, fish, meat and whole cereals should contain all the necessary vitamins. It is probable that others may be discovered in the future.

Fluids—Water. Without water life is not possible. It is necessary for all body processes and forms an essential part of all body tissues. It is the means by which food is conveyed to the cells and waste is removed. Approximately 66 per cent. (two-thirds) of the body weight is made up of water. The elimination of water plays a vital part in the regulation of body temperature. Our sources of water come from the fluid we drink, from the so-called solid food we eat, which in many cases is largely water, and from the oxidation of food in our tissue cells. Our intake of fluid must replace that constantly being excreted from the body, and in health we require between four to five pints (app. 3,000 ccs.) daily from all sources. A person who is ill often requires rather more than this, approximately six to seven pints daily (app. 4,000 ccs.). A healthy person should drink about two pints a day (app. 1,080 ccs.). Fortunately, our water requirements are to some extent controlled by our feeling of thirst. It must be remembered that if abnormal amounts of fluid are being lost by perspiration, salt is being lost as well and should be made up by taking small quantities of common salt. Stokers suffering from salt depletion get severe abdominal cramp. It is equally important to remember that the kidneys can only excrete certain quantities of salt and, therefore, it can be dangerous to drink abnormal amounts of salt water.

Flavoured drinks have very little food value unless milk and sugar are added. Tea and coffee are stimulating and refreshing, but should not be taken when the body is prepared for sleep. Fresh fruit juices, etc., are popular and good—they not only encourage people to drink plenty but, if properly prepared, should provide a valuable source of minerals and Vitamin C. Even so, providing the water on supply is safe and clean, people should be encouraged to drink it when thirsty.

Roughage. This consists mainly of cellulose from carbohydrate foods, vegetables and fruit, and to a less extent animal foods. Roughage forms bulk in the intestines, and while it is probably an asset because it stimulates peristalsis, it is not proved to be an essential. Milk, which contains no roughage, is the natural food for babies.

METABOLISM—AND A WELL-BALANCED DIET

This is the term used to describe the activity which goes on in the tissues when simple food substances which have been absorbed are broken down and used to form new cells. This activity creates heat and energy. As a result of these activities waste products are produced which must be eliminated by the excretory organs of the body. *Metabolism* can be said to consist of two processes: Katabolism, which is the breaking down of substances and tissue cells, and Anabolism, which is the building up of new tissue cells from chemical substances derived from digested foods.

This activity is going on continuously in our bodies, during sleeping as well as waking hours, but the rate of it varies with individuals and with different conditions. In the individual it is probably age, size and activity which influences metabolism most, activity being mainly controlled by the hormones produced by glands, particularly thyroxin from the thyroid gland. The conditions affecting metabolism are climate and the type of work the individual has to do. Cold climates and muscular exertion increase metabolism.

While it may be thought that during sleep and rest metabolism stops, this is not so. In fact, quite a lot of activity is going on to maintain the function of the various vital body systems. For instance, the heart and blood vessels are active maintaining the blood circulation; the respiratory system and the urinary system must go on working. To some extent the digestive system is functioning as well. All these systems require sugar and oxygen to create muscle activity, and about half the daily number of calories are required during rest as compared to the amount used when the body is active. The term *Basal Metabolic Rate* (B.M.R.) is used to describe the rate at which the body uses fuel, in other words, the rate of metabolism, while at complete rest, twelve hours after taking food. This rate may be estimated by measuring with special apparatus the amount of oxygen inhaled and the amount of carbon dioxide exhaled. The size, weight and age of the subject must be taken into account. A special chart is required and the rate expressed in the number of calories. For an adult man the rate is approximately 1,800 Calories, for a woman 1,500 Calories.

OBESITY

Obesity exists when a person is ten per cent more than normal weight according to height, age and sex. Child obesity has replaced malnutrition as a major problem in child health. Unfortunately there is some evidence to suggest that it is becoming more prevalent among adults. Not only does this cause the individual to be a greater health risk but it is a physical disability which predisposes to a number of diseases such as hypertension, heart and liver disease, and diabetes. Excessive weight aggravates joint problems such as osteo arthritis and causes other complications. Obesity influences morbidity and mortality rates adversely and in addition causes a great deal of loneliness and unhappiness.

Although obesity is seen among children and the chances are that these will become obese adults, it is more often a problem of middle and later years and affects both men and women. Occasionally an endocrine imbalance may be responsible but it is more often due to habitual or emotional overeating. The former—habitual overeating—may be due to family custom, sociability etc. and most emotional overeating is the result of boredom, loneliness and unhappiness.

Emotional overeating may be associated with other problems suggesting social and emotional maladjustment such as pilfering. The individual hungry for approval and affection finds satisfaction in overeating.

From every point of view it is important to control weight by attention to diet—particularly it is vital to avoid eating between meals, to avoid getting hungry and then eating large meals. To choose the right kind of food avoiding excessive carbohydrates and to make every effort to attack underlying causes and to take plenty of exercise.

To maintain normal weight one must balance energy intake (food) with energy output (activity). To lose weight one must increase activity and reduce food intake. Incentives are sometimes valuable, the greatest encouragement is the approval of family and friends and the ability to buy fashionable clothes at reasonable cost.

POSTURE, EXERCISE AND RECREATION

Posture. Physical education should form an important part in the school curriculum. Good posture is related to positive health. By posture is meant the position or bearing of the body; and, if the bony structure of the body is normal, and the individual is fit, this should give an impression of alertness and general well-being. When standing the head should be held up, the shoulders back, chest expanded, the abdomen and buttocks tucked in, with both feet firmly on the ground. Walking should be smooth and easy with arms free, head held high, and good foot movements used. The sitting position is equally important. The body weight should be borne by the pelvis and not the lower part of the spine, shoulders kept well back and head well up. Good posture allows proper ventilation of the lungs and enables joints and internal organs to function in their natural position. Good habitual posture is a social grace that is an advantage and should be encouraged from an early age.

Defects of posture due to bad habits of standing and sitting should be investigated, and individual help and corrective treatment given to those needing it. One must also remember, however, that these defects may be due to bad conditions of work, unsuitable furniture, poor lighting, fatigue, lack of sleep, debility or actual disease. Well-fitting, comfortable shoes and clothing are also important.

Slight curvature of the spine, flat feet, round shoulders, poking head are common defects.

Physical Exercise. Together with fresh air, sunlight, food, warmth and rest, exercise plays a vital part in the maintenance of positive health. It is particularly important in the growing child. Physical exercise is stimulating and should make the body experience a feeling of well-being. Naturally, the extent of the exercise must be suitable to the age of the individual. Physical exercise requires muscle activity which, in turn, demands greater supplies of oxygen and sugar, and results in the creation of heat. This extra heat produced is dissipated by the extra sweat evaporated from the surface of the body.

The demands made by the muscles for more oxygen and sugar stimulate the respiratory and cardio-vascular systems, generally speeding up activity and so increasing the ventilation of the lungs and improving the blood circulation throughout the body. This stimulation enables the brain to work more efficiently, and increases the general resistance of the body to disease. Proper ventilation of the lungs discourages the occurrence of respiratory infections.

From babyhood upwards exercise should form a regular part of the daily programme. Little children are rarely still and should get plenty in the ordinary process of natural play, but part of the exercise each day is best taken out of doors. Suitable clothing should be provided which is warm and comfortable, and shoes that are well fitting, well supporting and that keep the feet dry.

School programmes of children and adolescents should be so arranged as to provide adequate breaks for exercise, some of which should be taken out of doors regardless of the weather.

As one grows older, exercise is still important, and becomes no less important with the elderly. The retired man or woman who can remain active and enjoy daily exercise is so much better for it. A hobby, such as gardening, walking or golf, is very valuable.

Exercise becomes no less important when an individual is confined to bed, or one part of the body is immobilised in plaster. Controlled active or passive exercises are taught by the physiotherapists to keep the muscles in tone, and stimulate the circulation. Breathing exercises are given to ventilate the lungs.

Mental Exercise. Like other body tissues the brain cells thrive best when they are properly used. A squinting child will, in time, lose the sight of the so-called lazy eye if it is allowed to go on being lazy. This is because the acutely sensitive nervous collection of cells called the retina, which is the termination of the optic nerve, will gradually diminish in sensitivity and in time become useless. This happens because the cells have not been stimulated and used. The same is true of other body structures.

Small children usually get plenty of mental exercise. They are learning to do many things for the first time, to crawl and walk and talk, all most complex procedures requiring a good deal of mental and physical co-ordination. They are hearing and seeing new things and beginning to use all their special senses. During this period of rapid mental growth we must see that plenty of rest is possible.

Mental exercise continues spontaneously through the toddler stage and school years. Parents and teachers can best help by allowing children to think for themselves, to do things for themselves, and to work out their own problems. Parental help and advice should always be there, but how thwarting it is to an intelligent child who is enjoying working out a good jigsaw puzzle if a grown-up comes along and finds all the difficult pieces! A child with the right attitude towards learning will not have to be forced to exercise his brain. Force will only tend in most cases to affect the child adversely. The difficulties which have resulted from anxious parents driving their children to reach the standard for grammar school selection are only too well known.

All grades of intelligence need mental exercise. It is the aim of our present system to give everyone a basic education, so that the opportunities available for further study may be fully used.

It used to be said that the peak of one's mental receptive life occurred between the ages of twenty and thirty. This is no longer believed. If one's brain is kept exercised within individual normal limits, it goes on being just as receptive well into the period of middle age, and probably in some cases into the last decade of life.

Mental exercise is healthy and good and should be encouraged in all ways possible.

Recreation. The need for recreation begins when a child is small and continues, to some extent, all through life. The dictionary's definition of this word is interesting. Recreate means to refresh, revive, reanimate, to delight; and recreation is the process of being recreated, amused and refreshed after toil. However interesting and absorbing our work may be, we all need refreshing. If we deny ourselves recreation we become stale and tired and boring to our colleagues, and probably difficult to work and live with.

Recreation may take many forms, and may involve mental or physical exercise. The young child in the home or the nursery school is provided with toys which will satisfy his individual imagination and creativeness. Bricks, plasticine, paper, crayons and paints, toys on wheels and teddy bears are all necessary for indoor play, while open spaces free from danger, with sand, water, buckets, swings, seesaws and trees or climbing apparatus are all needed for the toddler out of doors. Suitable clothes which are comfortable, warm enough and not too costly to replace, are necessary if this form of recreation is to be really enjoyed.

The child at day or boarding school is usually well catered for with regard to recreation. In most schools a certain amount of regular mental or physical recreation forms part of the day's programme, but quite a lot is often left to the child's own choice. All forms of sport, swimming, dancing, drama, music, painting, reading, should be available. This is not only to provide the necessary exercise and recreation, but as part of a wider general education, which teaches a child to use his leisure time in a constructive way, so that when he grows beyond school years he will be able to enjoy his life fully.

The enjoyment of participation in any form of social or recreational clubs, if well organised, is useful, not only as recreation but in helping to form the character of the adolescent.

After school years, physical and mental hobbies started in childhood years may be carried on. After marriage, the family usually keeps both parents busy, and recreation is taken in a way that the whole family may enjoy. When the children are fully grown, old hobbies may be revived or fresh ones cultivated, and the Local Authorities of this country provide a wealth of recreational facilities to suit all tastes.

REST, SLEEP AND FATIGUE

Rest and relaxation are essential needs of all human beings. Individual needs vary, but all the systems of the body require a period of rest every twenty-four hours. The young child up to three or five years old needs a rest some time during the daytime. It is not necessary that he should sleep, but he should relax and stretch out on a comfortable bed with plenty of fresh air, preferably out of doors. The muscular, digestive and nervous systems all benefit. Mental and emotional rest in an adult is particularly important, and is probably best provided by a complete change of activity.

All growing children and adults who have suffered illness need more rest than ordinary healthy adults. Insufficient rest decreases immunity to disease, and may precipitate ill-health or cause mental fatigue. Rest and relaxation are closely linked with recreation.

Noise Control.—Florence Nightingale once said, " Unnecessary noise is the most cruel absence of care which can be inflicted on either sick or well". In recent years the world has become a noisy place, and is fast becoming noisier. A hundred years ago our grandparents were horrified by the noise of a steam train; now that is not so, most of us like it, but we are equally horrified by the noise of a jet plane. In time we shall no doubt become accustomed to that.

Recently there have been many inquiries into noise—particularly into noise in hospital. It is generally agreed that noise is bad, it irritates and frays the nerves, but is often accepted with resignation.

To a sick person, or one concentrating on a particular task, it is the small repeated noise that can be so irritating. Creaking boards, tapping and squeaking shoes, rattling keys can all be very disturbing. Other noises such as a continuous background rumbling of traffic can hardly be noticed but the sudden roar of a motor bicycle is distressing.

In hospital much of the equipment can contribute to the noise: trolleys with squeaking wheels, or rattling shelves, screens, bed-curtains, door springs, oxygen cylinders. Noises from the kitchen are often excessive and disturbing, as are the noises of other patients snoring or mentally confused. Many mechanical noises, from water pipes, lifts, etc., must also be considered.

Tolerable noise level varies from one person to another. The control of noise in hospital depends on the co-operation of the nursing, administrative and maintenance personnel in minimising noise at its source by:

(a) isolating and muffling structure-borne reverberations caused by impact, by providing sound-reducing walls and floors between the sources of noise and the patients.

(b) applying absorbents to surfaces of areas where noise is likely to occur.

Noise and vibration nuisances—Control of noise in the community is in the hands of the local authority and noise and vibration complaints are investigated by community health inspectors.

There is a trend towards greater noise consciousness on the part of the public and this is particularly apparent where industrial and residential developments meet. Planning authorities must take this into account when considering permission for the establishment of airports and industrial plant in residential areas.

Some universities are undertaking research into the effects of sound and vibration.

Sleep. Sleep obviously provides the most perfect form of rest. It is a period when the metabolic processes of the body are slowed down so that a large proportion of its sources of energy are available for growth. Sleep probably provides the only form of complete mental rest. It is essential for a period each day. A new baby sleeps twenty hours a day and wakes only to feed. As he grows older he gradually stays awake longer and longer. The rate of mental and physical growth of a small child is tremendous. Although this continues through to adult years, there is a gradual diminution in the rate. There is an acceleration during the adolescent years, and it is unfortunate that the educational and social demands made on the adolescent are so heavy that the amount of sleep is often too much reduced.

The quality of sleep is as important as the quantity. It should be quiet, restful and undisturbed, providing complete physical and mental repose. This is best achieved in a single comfortable bed alone in a room. The bed should have a firm mattress, light warm bed-clothes and a small pillow. The bedroom should be well ventilated and reasonably quiet. Night clothes should be warm, lightweight and comfortable. The position in bed varies, and most individuals develop their own particular position. Providing the body is relaxed, the joints preferably slightly flexed and the breathing apparatus clear, it is satisfactory.

Children and adults should have the right attitude towards bed. Healthy children should like their beds, should go off to sleep quickly, wake up equally quickly and get quickly out of bed. Many things may interfere with a child's going to sleep: excitement, over-tiredness, disappointment, fear, cold feet or hunger. A happy contented mind, a suitable bedtime story, prayers and a goodnight kiss all help to make bedtime a very happy event, and sleep more assured. A favourite toy or teddy to cuddle in bed is also enjoyed by most children. It is generally believed that there is no justification in denying a child a safe night light, if he is genuinely frightened of the dark.

Much of the above applies equally to adults. Insomnia is so often due to an alert, troubled mind. The understanding, sympathetic night nurse, who will find time to listen to her patient's troubles, to make a hot soothing drink, ensure the patient's feet are warm, the bed comfortable, and the ward reasonably quiet, is invaluable. Indigestion and a full bladder may also interfere with sleep and should be avoided.

Individual needs for sleep vary a good deal. Persistent prolonged denial of individual needs leads to a reduced resistance to disease and lower mental efficiency. Arrears of sleep can and should be made up, provided conditions are suitable, at any time of the day.

There is no justification for the old saying " one hour before eleven is worth two after seven ".

The average amount of sleep required depending on age is:

Two years old: 14–16 hours a day; 1–2 hours of this may be spent during the latter part of the morning or early afternoon. To bed about 5 p.m.

Four years old: 12–14 hours a day. A period of rest, not necessarily sleep, during the afternoon is an advantage to both mother and child. To bed at 5 to 5.30 p.m.

Six to 8 years old: 11–12 hours a day. To bed at 6.30 to 7 p.m.

Eight to 11 years old: 10–11 hours a day. To bed at 7 to 7.30 p.m.

Twelve to 14 years old: 9–10 hours a day. To bed at 8 to 8.30 p.m.

Fourteen to 18 years old: 8–9 hours a day.

Adults require between 6 and 8 hours sleep.

Fatigue. There are many causes and manifestations of fatigue—physical, mental and psychological. It can be due to the condition of one system or of the whole body. The muscles of the healthy body will suffer from fatigue if they are over-stimulated, and a feeling described as cramp will occur. This painful sensation occurs if the muscles are demanding more oxygen than the blood can supply and the products of combustion are not carried away. The healthy brain will suffer fatigue if it is excessively over-stimulated. School children working for higher examinations may suffer from this. *Psychological fatigue* is the condition found in persons exhausted by movements that would not affect normal people, or those suffering from the boredom of repetitive movements such as are made in factories.

HABIT FORMATION

The capacity to form habits is inborn, and many habits are formed as a result of the inborn tendency of young children to mimic others, particularly their parents. A habit is defined as "an action at first requiring attention, which comes to be performed without attention if repeated sufficient times under similar conditions". There are habits of thought as well as of action. Good habits can be a tremendous asset. Their advantages may be thought out under the following headings: those that

(1) Save time and energy.

(2) Give social security.

(3) Are useful in an emergency.

(4) Help to maintain good health.

(5) Those habits of thought, study and work which do so much to bring about success.

Generally speaking, good habits are fairly easily learnt; so are bad habits. The best way to stop a bad habit is by putting a good one in its place.

While good habits are valuable, it is important not to allow oneself to be entirely controlled by habit. One who has become the slave of habit is " in a rut " and should have a change of occupation and surroundings. It is important to keep one's mind flexible and receptive to new ideas, and to realise that it may be necessary from time to time to change certain habits and cultivate new ones.

Habit training begins soon after birth. Those that influence health and happiness continue to be taught by parents and teachers in the home and school. Most are best taught by example, and the reasons why each is necessary must be sensible and understandable if the child queries its usefulness.

Some of the important habits which should be taught are:

(1) Bladder and bowel control, and regular convenient elimination.

(2) Sleep and rest.

(3) Dental care.

(4) Feeding and meal time behaviour.

(5) Those applied to the care of the skin, hair and nails.

(6) Those of dress and, when older, the use of cosmetics.

(7) Good manners and general courtesy.

(8) Good clean useful habits of thought. Unselfishness, thoughtfulness, kindness, honesty and trustworthiness.

When parents are discussing habit training in young children, with a nurse or teacher, it is important to remind them that although they may be anxious to teach their children to behave in a socially acceptable manner, it is wrong and even dangerous to try to force the formation of a habit beyond the child's capacity. The ages at which children develop vary considerably, and while habits may be encouraged they should never be forced. This applies particularly to bladder and bowel control.

Parents should realise that the most effective way to teach children to develop good health habits is to set them good examples.

GENERAL CLEANLINESS OF THE BODY

During this century we have all become much more germ-conscious and although one would not underestimate the importance of personal cleanliness, one must keep a sense of proportion, particularly where children are concerned. Children are not naturally clean and fond of soap and water, and see little sense in repeatedly being made to use it. Body cleanliness should be largely a matter of habit formation, it should not be forced or over-emphasised, and too much should not be expected at too early an age. It is good to see a happy energetic child, with grubby knees and hands, romping home ravenously hungry to the safety of happy parents. How much better this is than the picture of a child so clean and well dressed that he is afraid to play. One must, after all, take into account the facilities available before becoming too critical. It is easy to keep oneself and one's clothing clean if living in a modern house with all modern conveniences. How much more difficult it is to maintain high standards of cleanliness if living in less comfortable surroundings with no modern conveniences! Added to this, the family in such a position has probably a limited amount of money to spend on housekeeping. Nevertheless, cleanliness of the body is important. Children taught to appreciate this will grow up with good habits, will later become parents and will, in turn, teach their children the same good habits. Cleanliness of the body can be considered under the following headings:

(1) Cleanliness of the skin and its appendages.

(2) Cleanliness of the inside of the body.

(3) Mental cleanliness.

Cleanliness of the skin and its appendages. *The skin.*—Healthily functioning skin collects on its surface dried sweat, salt and grease and dried epithelial cells. This provides an ideal breeding ground for organisms that are naturally found on the skin as well as for those more dangerous. The decomposition of sweat and bacterial activity produces an unpleasant smell which may constitute a social nuisance. If skin in this condition is punctured or damaged in any way, organisms are more likely to penetrate the damaged tissues and set up infection. External parasites such as lice and the scabies mite are more likely to breed undisturbed. The natural pores in the skin get blocked and " blackheads " are more likely to occur—these may become infected. Because the pores are blocked sweat finds it difficult to escape to the surface of the body and evaporate. This, in turn, prevents the proper elimination of sweat and interferes to some extent with the temperature control of the body.

For all these reasons the skin should be washed each day with warm water and soap, and particular attention paid to parts where two skin surfaces lie in contact, and to parts richly supplied with sweat glands like the armpits and the groins. The easiest and most pleasant way to do this is to have a daily bath. Most mothers find it convenient to give the baby his daily bath in the morning before his ten o'clock feed. As he grows older, however, it is usual to give him his bath last thing at night before going to bed. If a bath is not possible the child can be washed with soap and water while standing in a basin. With children it is important to make the bath or wash-down enjoyable. It should be done in a warm room, the child protected from draughts, the water not too hot or too cold, and care taken not to let soap get into the child's eyes. Boats and toys which float on the water, and pretty sponges all help to make the bath something to look forward to. If water has to be heated on a stove or the tap water is very hot, particular care must be exercised to prevent babies and young children from getting scalded.

As children grow up and go to school they should learn to bath themselves, to wash behind their ears and knees, between their legs and between their toes. Careful and tactful parental supervision is necessary from time to time. Children should be taught to rinse the bath and handbasin when they have finished washing, to take the soap out of the water, shake out the flannel and hang up the towel to dry. Each child should have his own flannel and towel and both these should be frequently laundered.

After energetic sports a cold shower is stimulating and effective in ridding the skin of sweat and refreshing the body generally.

Most adults like to take their bath at night. A hot bath is sooth-ing but it should not be too hot. Those who like a bath in the morn-ing should have it warm or cold. The latter, if properly used, can be very invigorating and stimulating.

The hands need washing more frequently, but should not be excessively scrubbed or damaged by detergents or disinfectants. In cold weather they should be carefully dried. In the winter time suitable hand creams may be necessary to keep the skin supple and elastic. From an early age children should be taught to wash their hands *after* going to the lavatory and *before* sitting down to a meal. Adults should do the same and, in addition, should wash their hands before handling and preparing food. All public lavatories and cloak-rooms in institutions should provide suitable facilities to practise what is taught. Liquid soap and paper towels and electric hand driers are the most satisfactory. Where such facilities are not available clean or freshly laundered towels should be supplied. Unfortunately, many old public lavatories, and those in some old institutions, lack these facilities. To be effective the basin needs to be next to or very near the lavatory.

Cuts and abrasions on the skin should be cleansed and covered until they are healed.   Any inflamed or septic lesion should be carefully treated and kept covered. If on the hands, the utmost care should be taken when preparing or handling food, particularly if it is being prepared for infants and young children.

The skin on the feet may need special attention. Some people have a tendency to have perspiring feet and will therefore more easily develop an infection in between the toes—*tinea pedis* or " athlete's foot "—which causes the skin to become soggy and peel away, leaving raw painful patches. Because this is contagious it tends to affect families and may become a nuisance in boarding schools and institutions. This condition may also affect those whose feet do not perspire excessively. The best way to keep the skin between the toes healthy is to keep it clean and dry and, if necessary, use a proprietary powder specially for this condition. A daily change of socks and shoes is an advantage.

Elderly folk and those who suffer from diabetes mellitus must take particularly good care to keep their feet healthy and prevent any form of injury. Injury or danger signs such as colour change, discharge, swelling or throbbing should be treated medically.

A verruca is a simple wart which can occur on any part of the skin; that which occurs on the foot is called verruca pedis. It is thought to be caused by a virus infection and therefore tends to be acquired through use of communal showers, baths, swimming pools, etc. Verrucae can be painful and require proper treatment by a doctor or registered chiropodist.

Corns are small areas of very hard skin, varying in size from a small grain of rice to about the size of a pea. A hard clear or yellow centre is surrounded by hard skin and is the direct local response of the skin to pressure. Corns can be very painful and should be treated by a registered chiropodist.

Tanning of the skin is caused by the sun's rays. When naked skin is exposed to bright sunlight it reddens and may burn. If exposure is prolonged or burning excessive the person may exhibit signs of malaise,—headache, fever, and nausea. Fair skin is more sensitive than dark and great care needs to be taken not to risk exposing a baby's skin to excessive sun. When by the sea the cool wind blowing off the sea may disguise the actual strength of the sun which is at its strongest at midday. As tanning of the skin progresses, melanin, which is the normal colouring matter of the skin, increases. Dark races are born with a large amount of this pigment while white races have very little naturally.

Frost bite is equally damaging to the skin and is caused by prolonged and excessive chilling. On no account should frost bitten skin be warmed by artificial means. The circulaton should be stimulated and restored by energetic rubbing.

The Nails.—These should be kept clean, short and rounded. The cuticles should be soft and pushed well back and not allowed to crack. Care should be taken not to damage the cuticle by the too energetic use of a metal nail file. Children's nails should be very gently cleaned and cut without hurting. Toe nails should be kept clean and short, and should be cut straight and not rounded. Cuticles are best kept soft using a hand cream, and pushed gently back. If the toe nails are tending to grow into the tissues at the side it may help to cut a small V in the centre.

Well kept finger nails are not only beautiful but necessary for the full use of fingers. The habit of nailbiting, which is ordinarily associated with tension, not only spoils the look of the hands but endangers the health of the individual through the introduction of dirt and bacteria into the mouth.

The Hair.—Small babies should have their hair washed each day when bathed, but as the child gets older, from about 9 months upwards, it is usual to shampoo the hair once a week. A good brushing of the scalp is stimulating and gives the hair a glossy well-cared-for appearance. A soft brush is best for babies and young children. This can be changed gradually for one with harder bristles as the child gets older. Except in very cold and wet weather, the hair is best exposed to the fresh air. Hair is best worn, for little girls, in attractive hair styles, the modern " pony tail " or plaits if it is long, which is most attractive in small children if tied over the head. Short hair is best carefully shaped so that it does not become a nuisance to the child at school. Regular shampooing should be carried out with great care, to avoid making it unpleasant by allowing soap to get into the child's eyes, brushing or combing too vigorously, or using unpleasantly hot or cold water.

Some children's skins are naturally greasy, and the hair contains " dandruff ". This condition will usually improve if a spirit or soapless type of shampoo is used. As children grow older they should be taught how to wash their brushes and combs, and to do so regularly before washing the hair. Complaints of irritation or any suspicious scratching noticed at home or in school should be investigated. It may be due to infestation with pediculi. If this is the case, the head should be quietly and properly dealt with without fuss. It is probably a wise gesture to inform the school teacher by letter in case other children in the class are similarly affected. If the mother does not know how to treat the head, the Health Visitor will give advice, or the child's head could be treated at the school clinic.

Cleanliness of the Inside of the Body.   *The Mouth and Teeth.*—The mouth of a healthy baby is moist, pink and clean, and should not be interfered with in any way. If the baby is feverish and the mouth tends to be dry, it is still unwise to attempt to clean it by artificial means. A little extra cool boiled water given after or in between feeds is most effective. The most important point with regard to the cleanliness of the baby's mouth is that mother should see that all things likely to go into his mouth are reasonably clean. Food and bottle teats should be kept especially clean and toys and hands which may be sucked should be frequently washed. By about the age of two the child may be taught to use a small soft toothbrush and a pleasant toothpaste, and will soon develop the habit of brushing his teeth night and morning, if his parents set him a good example. It is most important that this procedure is not forced at too early an age. Children who are a little unwell should be encouraged to drink plenty of water or fruit juice. It is the most effective way of keeping the mouth clean. Everyone, especially toddlers and small children, should be encouraged to chew crusts and apples, and discouraged from eating sweets or starchy food immediately before going to bed.

Mouth cleanliness should be encouraged throughout childhood, and all children taken for regular visits to the dentist. Properly handled by the dentist and the parents, the child will grow to accept dental attention without fear. This habit created in childhood will usually continue through the adult years. Excellent advice is given to children in the school dental clinics. A toothbrush that is only moderately hard is advised. Brushing should be upwards, downwards, backwards and forwards on both sides, so that the teeth are cleaned on all surfaces; and the toothbrush should be periodically renewed.

In spite of energetic efforts to educate children and parents it is salutary to know that in the United Kingdom the number of tooth brushes bought annually is small compared to the population. The British Dental Association keeps the picture constantly under review and reports such information as nine million tooth brushes purchased in a country of fifty five million people. Some children lose all their deciduous teeth due to decay before the age of six. There is a long waiting list for false teeth with resulting nutritional effects.

It is suggested that fluoridation of water supply* is the quickest remedy, but, we could attack the cause of symptoms by reducing carbohydrate consumption, i.e. eating less biscuits, sweets, crisps, chocolates and by consuming less soft drinks. It has even been suggested that a tax on these commodities might be effective in diminishing the amount children eat and drink.

It is known that dental decay is an endemic disease of civilised communities initiated by the uncontrolled intake of refined carbo-hydrates and poor oral hygiene.

Nose and Ears.—The apertures of the nose and the ears are lined with delicate ciliated epithelium specially adapted for its position. Although in the past it has been taught that it is beneficial to clean out these orifices when bathing the baby and young child, most pædia-tricians now say it is unnecessary, many will go further and strongly advise against it. This applies particularly to the ears. The cilia of the aural passage will pass out wax to the external opening where it can be carefully removed without poking anything inside the passage. This applies equally to adults. Care should be taken not to introduce soap suds into the orifice which may get pushed down the passage by the towel or flannel, and get dried and mixed up with the natural cerumen. If the external meatus does get really blocked with wax then medical attention should be obtained.

With the nose, the natural sensitivity will cause a sneeze or the desire to blow the nose. Children should be taught to use a handker-chief properly, to hold one nostril and blow gently, then to do the same on the other side. Great care should be taken with small children not to hurt or pinch the nose when wiping it, and to provide the child with a pocket where he can keep his own handkerchief. The handkerchief should be changed for a clean one each day, and more often if the child has a cold. With a severe cold, paper hand-

* See page 47.

kerchiefs that can be destroyed are an advantage. A dirty handkerchief can be a serious source of infection not only to the owner but also to other people.

Intestinal Cleanliness.—If good habits of evacuation are started when a child is small, constipation should not occur. Every effort should be made to ensure that there is no reason why the child should dislike going to the lavatory. He may be frightened of the dark if there is no proper lighting. The seat may be too big so that he is afraid of falling in. The lavatory may be dirty or may smell unpleasantly or perhaps the routine is badly arranged so that there is not time to go. A routine allowing sufficient time to go to the lavatory after breakfast is the most useful habit to adopt. It is particularly convenient when the child starts school. For small children it is much better to continue to use a comfortable safe pot, and let the child gradually learn to use the grown-up lavatory. No undue attention should be taken if a small child has minor lapses of routine, or an occasional accident; and periodic attacks of constipation should not give rise to undue parental concern. If, however, there is concern, the child should not be made aware of it. Attention to the diet, which should include rather more roughage, plenty of fresh fruit and adequate amounts of water to drink, should counteract occasional constipation. Plenty of exercise and fresh air are also advised. If constipation is really worrying and persistent, then something mild such as a teaspoonful of red-label Petrolagar may help, but great care should be taken to avoid the necessity for regular use of laxatives or aperients.

The same advice is suitable for adults, although the causes of constipation may be, in addition to those mentioned above, such pathological conditions as hæmorrhoids, fissure or more serious complaints. With both children and adults, if the simple measures mentioned are not effective and constipation is causing concern, then medical advice should be sought.

All lavatories should be well ventilated and kept clean. Children should be taught to use them properly and so help to keep them so. Provision should be made for hand washing.

Special Points of Body Cleanliness with particular reference to the adolescent.

Menstruation.—A young girl who is menstruating usually gets proper instruction and advice from her mother. Nowadays most children are prepared for the event before it actually starts, but there are still some girls who have to find out for themselves, or who have parents with rather old-fashioned ideas. Some parents may tell their daughters it is dangerous to take a bath when menstruating. There is no scientific reason for this belief, in fact it is an advantage to have a warm bath, and it is certainly cleansing and refreshing. While menstruating, if it is not possible to have a daily bath, the groins and vulva should be washed thoroughly each day; a little talcum powder is a refreshing luxury, but not an essential. Sanitary pads should be changed regularly and disposed of properly. Girls should be taught to wrap the pad in waste paper or a specially provided bag, and then to burn it as soon as convenient. In schools, factories and institutions incinerators or sanibins are provided. Sanibins should be kept clean and covered, should be placed inside the lavatory; and incinerators should be as near as possible. Like washing basins, they will not be used unless well placed. Insoluble types should not be put down the lavatory. During menstruation a frequent change of pants should be encouraged.

While it is beyond the subject of body cleanliness, about which this chapter is concerned, one must mention the need to encourage the right outlook. All the old-fashioned terms such as " out of sorts ", " poorly ", " not well ", were so wrong—they are still sometimes used, and no wonder young girls tend to grow up with the idea that they should feel unwell while they are menstruating. They may be told to take things quietly, go by bus rather than walk, and all these things tend to suggest that the child does not feel well. The young girl who suffers least from dysmenorrhœa* is the one who behaves absolutely normally while menstruating, plays games, cycles, walks, baths, in fact does all the usual things without anyone being aware of the fact that she is menstruating. Many young girls will ask if they can swim and the proper use of Tampax may make this per-missable, otherwise one does not give permission because of other people swimming in the same water.

The Use of Tampax. Tampax is a soft surgical cotton wool plug specially shaped to slip into the vagina, to absorb the flow of blood during the menstrual period. It is used as an alternative to the sanitary pad. Two sizes are prepared, " Regular " and " Super ", the latter may be necessary for the first day when the flow is heavier, but the " Regular " size is adequate for most people.

Many young girls will ask if it is wise and safe to use Tampax and if it is necessary to seek medical advice before doing so. Many

* Note. Dysmenorrhoea—painful and difficult menstruation.

parents find it difficult to give advice unless they have themselves had experience of using them. Tampax is easy and safe to use provided one knows how—with each pack simple instructions are given. Unmarried girls can generally use them as effectively as married women. If any difficulty is encountered, and it may be in rare cases, then medical advice should be obtained. It is most important to change them regularly and to be particularly careful to remove the last one used at the end of the menstrual flow. Failure to do this is sometimes the cause of vaginal discharge. Women going abroad to live in the hot countries are advised to use Tampax in preference to the conventional sanitary pad.

Sweating in the Axillae and Body Odour.—Body odour should not normally occur if the skin is kept clean and clothes washed or cleaned frequently, but many girls are troubled by excessive perspiration. This particularly affects the adolescent who is inclined to be nervous, and especially the girl who gets excited. Excessive sweating under the arms is not only embarrassing, but is also expensive, it ruins clothes. Some parents still tell their daughters that deodorants and anti-perspirants are dangerous. Unfortunately, cheap and unreliable deodorants may cause skin trouble and a good anti-perspirant may cause irritation if it is not used properly.

The unpleasant smell of body odour is caused by the decomposition of sweat and by bacterial action, the latter particularly if there is a growth of hair. Sweat allowed to decompose in woollen material is particularly offensive. Shaving under the arms, if carefully done with a clean sharp safety razor, is not dangerous. The regular use of a good anti-perspirant, used with the maker's instructions, is most effective—it may not stop perspiration entirely but it does limit it considerably. If perspiration is sufficiently excessive to cause serious continued distress an operation can be done which will control it.

Boys and Girls who suffer from Blackheads and Acne.—This is a fairly common condition among adolescents. It particularly affects those with a greasy type of skin. The pore from the sebaceous gland becomes blocked with sebum, and a hard head forms on the top. This is called a comedo. Infection may occur under the top.

This type of skin needs to be kept very clean. Regular washing is necessary using a good soap, hot water and a flannel; this must be followed by careful rinsing and drying. Exposure of the skin to fresh air and sunlight is good, especially the latter. Evacuation of the blocked pore is advised, providing only gentle pressure is used and the skin not badly squeezed and damaged. There is a very useful little instrument, the *comedo remover*, sold by surgical instrument makers and many chemists. Blackheads should be removed before they get too big. Sweets and carbohydrate foods should be limited and attention paid to matters such as sufficient sleep, fresh air, exercise and avoidance of constipation. Men are often helped by changing from ordinary to electric razors.

Fortunately acne rarely persists beyond the early twenties; if it does, medical attention should be obtained.

Mental Cleanliness. A good clean healthy outlook on life has its beginnings in early childhood. Intelligent healthy children are naturally curious and inquisitive, and from an early age will begin to ask questions. All children's questions should be simply and honestly answered, and in most cases, even if the answer is not fully understood, it will be dismissed from the child's mind. Giving young children the opportunity to have animals as pets, letting them grow up with simple knowledge about mating, will usually make things very much easier. By far the best and safest way for children to find out about life is in this way and from their own parents and home. The best way to give a child wrong ideas and force him to go to his school friends for information—which will probably be a bit distorted anyhow—is to make a mystery of such things. The amount of good teaching that goes on in most schools nowadays on biology and hygiene is very helpful.

From an early age children can be encouraged to think good of their neighbour, to be kind and thoughtful to others less fortunate, unselfish, appreciative, honest and helpful at home; to be courteous to everyone and kindly and helpful, especially to elderly folk or those in any way disabled. Membership of all the good Youth Organisations, Cubs, Brownies, Guides, Scouts, Sunday School, Red Cross and St. John and many other activities give opportunities for strengthening this good type of mental outlook.

As children grow older they will learn to look for, and appreciate, more senior types of clubs. As their education advances they will learn to be selective in their reading, viewing of television and listening to wireless programmes.

The well-educated maturing adolescent has learnt what is good, can see and read about the good side of life as well as the sordid, and will have learnt to steer a middle course. Having satisfied his curiosity he will, in most cases, be no longer interested. Behind all this mental growth and development, the parents play a tremendously important role by quietly influencing their children mainly by example and encouragement.

Children at school will sometimes hear new words which they think are either rude or swear words. They will produce such words at home just to see the effect, and if it produces anger or alarm they will think it is something really worth knowing. If, on the other hand, it is completely ignored or just answered naturally without fuss, the whole thing falls flat and there is then no point in the child's mind of doing it again. He might perhaps repeat it two or three times, but if still no notice is taken he will forget all about it. Naturally, if parents use undesirable language and fail to practise good manners to their children and themselves, then no one can blame the children for doing the same.

Temperament and character, strengthened by conscience, are the result of successfully growing up. Once temperament and character are firmly established between the age of twenty and thirty they do not appreciably alter.

A human being thus well matured cannot help to affect this fellow men profoundly. He has all that is good for building his own family on sure foundations and shaping his own life for the good of the community as a whole.

CHOICE AND CLEANLINESS OF CLOTHING AND FOOTWEAR

Clothing. Clothes are necessary to assist in the regulation of body temperature, and to protect it from injury. They are also worn to satisfy an existing need to conform to a particular social pattern.

In choosing clothes the following points should be considered:

(1) Whether they are required to conserve the body heat, or to protect the body from a source of outside heat—in other words to keep the body cool.

(2) Whether they are required to stand up to excessive wear and tear—durability.

(3) Whether they are easily washable, or in some cases able to be cleaned.

(4) Whether they look attractive.

(5) Whether they are comfortable to wear.

(6) With children's clothes especially, it is important to consider whether the material is particularly inflammable.

(7) The amount of money one has to spend.

On the whole, clothing to-day is relatively simple compared with that of our grandparents' time. This applies especially to underclothes.

Choice of the right clothing, and of sufficient amount, minimises the strain on the heat regulating centre of the brain. Intelligent adjustment to suit the weather conditions is important.

Damp clothes, whether wet from rain or perspiration, should be changed immediately. Not only are they uncomfortable but, if allowed to dry on the body will cause excessive chilling of the body. This applies particularly if dried by a strong wind.

The choice of materials for clothes is important. Lightweight loosely woven materials which trap plenty of air are naturally bad conductors of heat, and so are used to conserve the body heat. Pure wool is best in this respect, but, unfortunately, it tends to shrink and may irritate the skin. Cellular materials are good and much used for children's and adults' underclothes. Pure silk is also a good conductor of heat, but it does not absorb moisture well, and is very expensive. It is quite effective for warm underclothes and night wear. Linen is excellent as bed linen, but does not absorb moisture like cotton.

A variety of manmade (synthetic) materials are now available. They trap air around the body and are therefore very warm but do not absorb moisture. They need frequent and careful washing, are relatively inexpensive and durable. Many new synthetic fibres are constantly coming on to the market, many are combined with cotton and/or wool and all seem to be strong and effective.

Artificial silk is cool and is still used a good deal for underclothes. It is inexpensive. Flannelette is *not good* for clothing, although it is inexpensive. It is not very warm and is *inflammable* and a danger to children.

Cotton is good in warm weather. It easily absorbs perspiration and quickly dries, so cooling the body. It is reasonably inexpensive and fairly easy to wash.

The materials mentioned above are those most suitable for underclothes. Most children's underclothes consist nowadays of vest and pants. Outer clothes of various colours may be of any of the materials mentioned above. In addition fur, leather, Terylene, plastic and rubber are all used for outer clothing to keep out the wind and rain, but materials that do not allow ventilation are apt to be uncomfortable if worn for very long.

The choice of colours for clothing is important. White and light colours are cool, whereas darker colours, particularly red and black, are warm.

The design of clothes is also important. Those for little children should be loose and well fitting, preferably hung from the shoulder. They should be easy to put on and take off. Any necessary elastic, such as that in panties, should be sufficiently wide to be comfortable and not too tight. Equally they should not be too loose. School woven pants of a dark colour are probably best worn with a white cellular pair for a lining. For economic reasons design should be simple and the material such that it will stand up to frequent washing. In warm and moderate weather it is best to leave the arms and legs and head uncovered and provide a loose woolly jacket or sweater for cooler periods.

In colder and wet weather, however, cover for the legs and arms and some form of comfortable hat are required. This applies particularly to little children. For play in cold weather they are probably happiest in tough dungarees made of corduroy or denim, with some type of jersey or windcheater and tights underneath.

In the summer by the seaside very little clothing is required, except when the sun is really hot. When it is, protection should be given to the skin until it has become sufficiently tanned to stand the sun. Some children with sensitive fair skins will always need some form of protection. Particular precautions should be taken if the heat of the sun is masked by a cool sea breeze.

Underclothing, particularly, should be changed and washed regularly—at least once a week.

Girls and boys as they grow older should learn to choose their own clothes, be educated in the fashions available, allowed to develop their own styles and choose their own colours to suit their personalities and should learn to care for their clothes and appreciate their value. A clothing allowance for the developing adolescent is a valuable aid in this respect.

Probably the most effective teaching is that taught by teachers and parents who set a good example.

Footwear. Comfortable feet are so important that every effort should be made from an early age to keep them in good condition. Providing there is nothing dangerous on the floor, little children are very happy to run around bare-footed. Socks and shoes, when worn, should be of the right size and not too heavy. Socks should be changed and washed frequently, and both socks and shoes discarded as soon as they are no longer big enough. Shoes should be comfortable, strong and weatherproof and suitable for the time of the year. If feet are inclined to sweat it is best to alternate shoes each day so that they have an opportunity to dry completely. In between wearing they should be left in the circulating air. Heels and soles should be even and well cared for, and the size and shape of the shoe should suit the individual foot. They should advisably be at least half an inch larger than the feet. Flat feet and other foot deformities may be hereditary or due to the wearing of faulty shoes. During wet weather Wellington boots are probably the most satisfactory. These are most comfortable worn with loosely fitting woollen socks. Children should be taught the necessity of changing shoes and stockings if the feet are wet, and it is good training to teach them to leave off their outdoor shoes for lighter ones when in school and at home. Appropriate shoes should be worn for physical training and all different types of games.

Adolescent girls are often tempted to buy fashionable shoes which are bad for the feet. Any shoes which cramp the toes or tend to push the weight of the body too much on to the toes will cause corns, hammer toes and other deformities.

PARASITES AND VERMIN—PREVENTIVE MEASURES AND DISINFESTATION

A parasite is some form of animal or plant life which lives in or upon another, drawing nutriment directly from it. The body providing the nutriment is usually referred to as the host. In this chapter it is intended only to deal with the more common parasites which affect personal health and happiness, e.g., body lice and intestinal worms.

Vermin can be described as living things which will cause harm to crops, animals and man. Again, only those commonly affecting personal health will be dealt with in this chapter.

In the past, parasites and vermin have been responsible for spreading disease, for causing famine by destroying food and, in many cases, have shaped the outcome of wars. Nowadays, apart from typhus fever carried by lice and bubonic plague by rat fleas, there is little evidence of their causing disease; but, despite a high standard of personal and communal health, verminous conditions among school children and vagrants still present quite a problem. Every effort is made by the school health service and the Local Authorities to prevent and destroy breeding grounds, to treat and cleanse infested persons and teach personal cleanliness. Housing conditions are improved and vermin destroyed in ports and warehouses. Unfortunately, in spite of this, infestation is often a family affair, and unless all the members of the family will co-operate, reinfestation will occur. Fortunately, we now have the advantage of a wide variety of chemical substances, relatively easy to use and very effective.

Internal Animal Parasites. *Nematodes. Thread Worm (oxyuris vermicularis).*—This is probably the most common of the intestinal worms in the United Kingdom and very common indeed in less developed countries. Children are mainly affected. The worms inhabit the cæcum and rectum, and appear like fine white threads in the fæces. The female worms tend to migrate to the anus at night; they lay their eggs around the anus and buttocks giving rise to intense irritation. This causes restlessness, sleeplessness, enuresis and, in some cases, convulsions. Unfortunately, as a result of the irritation, the child scratches and gets his fingers infected with the ova. In this way he reinfests himself. Because he is restless he tends to suck his fingers and so the life cycle starts again. The thread worm eggs are often found on underwear, nightwear, bedding, towels, lavatory seats and so on. They are very small and light and float in the air particularly when clothing are removed and shaken. The eggs can also get into household dust which is a further source of infection.

Infestation in the first instance is caused by food or drinking water infested with the ova. Once infested, every effort should be made to prevent the child reinfesting himself. Hands should be kept very clean and nails short. Flannel and towel should be kept separate and frequently boiled. Night clothes and bed linen should be frequently changed—pyjamas are probably the best form of night attire—and boilable gloves can be worn. Bathing and thorough washing every morning will remove any threadworm eggs deposited on the body during the night. Some form of mercurial ointment smeared around the anus will kill the migrating worms and lessen the irritation. The most simple curative treatment advised nowadays is gentian violet capsules or Pripsen* granules given by mouth, but any treatment such as this must be under medical control. For complete eradication of thread worm infestation success is more likely when each member of the household takes a single dose of Pripsen simultaneously.

Bedrooms and lavatories should be frequently cleaned and kept well aired. Threadworm eggs die more quickly in cool dry air.

The Round Worm (ascaris lumbricoides).—This large worm looks

* Pripsen is piperozine phosphate with senna.

very like the ordinary earth worm, except that it is whitish-yellow in colour. It is most common in countries where sanitation is poor and the water supply unreliable. In this country children are mostly affected by drinking water, or eating food such as salads or raw vegetables, contaminated with the ova. If fertilised ova are swallowed

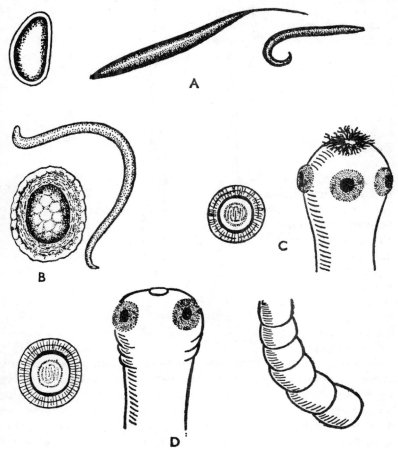

Fig. 18. Internal Animal Parasites.

A. Thread worm (*oxyuris vermicularis*). B. Round worm (*ascaris lumbricoides*). C. Pork tape worm (*tænia solium*). D. Beef tape worm (*tænia saginata*) (see text).

they develop into larvæ in the small intestine, pass through the blood stream to the liver, and then to the lungs. From the alveoli the larvæ migrate to the trachea and larynx to be swallowed into the stomach. In the stomach the larva develops and the worm inhabits the upper part of the small intestine. This causes irritation, nervous irritability and possibly anæmia. The fully developed worm may be passed per rectum or may occasionally be vomited. The male worm is about 4 to 8 in. long, the female slightly longer.

Prevention of this infestation is secured by a high standard of personal cleanliness, efficient food inspection and preparation, good sanitation and safe water supply. If infestation occurs medical treatment is required.

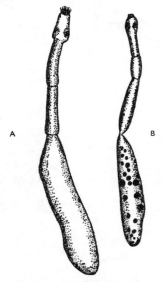

Fig. 19. Internal Animal Parasites.
Hydatid disease worm (echinococcus granulosus)
A. Incomplete parasite, showing head with hooklets and suckers.   B. Complete parasite showing scolex and three segments, the last one mature.

Cestodes.—These parasites are commonly known as tape worms. There are four main varieties, each having special characteristics. They vary in length from 10 to 30 ft. though the type causing hydatid disease is only about ¼ in. long. Each tape worm consists of a head and a varying number of segments. Each segment is hermaphroditic, i.e. possessing both male and female sexual organs. Each active segment is capable of producing large numbers of fertilised ova. The head of the tape worm is equipped with suckers and, in some cases, with hooks. As long as the head is attached to the intestinal wall more segments will develop—those segments farthest away from the head becoming progressively larger. As soon as the head is removed the rest of the worm will die. From time to time segments will break away and be found in the fæces into which large numbers of eggs are constantly discharged. The life story of the tape worm is complex—each must have more than one host to complete its life cycle.

Infestation by these worms can give rise to nervous irritability, anorexia or the reverse: a voracious appetite and possibly anæmia. Infestation is caused by diseased meat such as pork or beef, or fresh-water fish—in all instances food which has not been adequately cooked. Infestation may also occur through eating food handled by someone whose hands are contaminated by the ova.

Treatment under careful medical control is required. This aims at destroying the head of the worm and causing its expulsion. Prevention of reinfestation is important, careful personal cleanliness is necessary. Routine meat and fish inspection has done much to control this type of infestation.

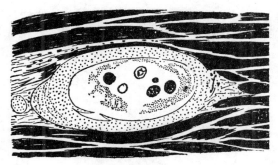

Fig. 20. Trichinosed muscle.
Trichinella embryo encysted in human muscle.

The four main types of tape worms are:

(1) Pork tape worm—*tænia solium*.

(2) Beef tape worm—*tænia mediocanellata (tænia saginata)*.

(3) Fish tape worm—*dibothriocephalus latus*.

(4) Hydatid disease worm—*tænia echinococcus (echinococcus granulosus)*. This worm is slightly different from the rest. It is smaller and uses man and sheep as the intermediate host. The infestation is passed on by dogs. In man large hydatid cysts form in the abdominal organs, mainly the liver, rather less often in the lung, occasionally in the brain.

A slender worm *trichina spiralis* has its larval stage in pork, and if the pork is eaten uncooked the larvæ settle in the muscles in large quantities causing *trichiniasis* with symptoms of swelling, muscle pains, fever and occasionally death.

External Parasites. *Lice (pediculi).*—There are three varieties of these wingless insects which infest human beings and suck their blood.

(1) The head louse—*pediculus capitis.* In spite of an improved standard of cleanliness this is still not an uncommon infestation among school children. The head louse is a small insect with three pairs of legs, each of which is equipped with claws. It lives on the scalp from which it sucks blood by means of a sucker protruding from its head. The female lays about four eggs a day—these are deposited on the hair close to the scalp. The eggs are attached

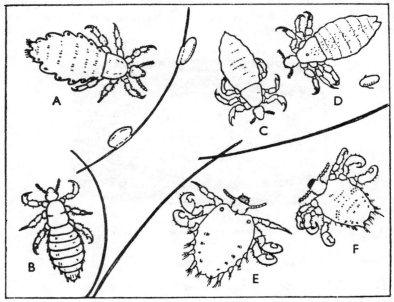

Fig. 21. External Parasites.
A. Head louse female (*pediculus capitis*). B. Male and eggs or nits on human hair. C. Body louse male (*pediculus vestimente*). D. Female and egg. E. Crab louse female (*phthirus pubis*). F. Male.

tightly to the hair by a form of cement. They appear white and shining and under ordinary conditions take about a week to hatch. The presence of head lice gives rise to itching and scratching. In the process of scratching, dirty finger nails often infect the skin, so giving rise to impetigo and swollen glands in the neck. Treatment is simple and effective. The old standard treatment with sassafras oil has been replaced by that of an emulsion of Dicophane B.P.C. This is smeared on to the hair, which is left for up to twenty-four hours, then washed and tooth-combed. The process is repeated in a week to kill hatching lice. The hairbrush, comb, towel, etc. and

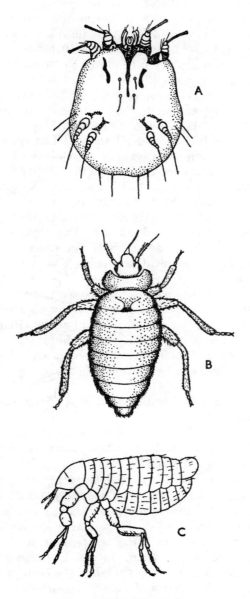

Fig. 22. External Parasites.
A. *Sarcoptes scabei.* B. Bed bug (*cimex lectularius*).
C. Flea (*pulex irritans*) (see text).

clothes should be washed after use. The pillow cases and bed linen should also be changed. After cleansing the head should be daily tooth-combed and inspected for a time until it is certain there is no further infestation. It is an interesting fact that head lice will leave the head of a person if the temperature rises to any extent, or if the temperature falls, as in death.

(2) The body louse—*pediculus corporis*. This insect is very similar in habit and appearance to the head louse. It bites the skin of the body and sucks blood in the same way. It lays its eggs along the seams and in the fold of underclothes. These eggs take about a week to hatch. Treatment is again simple and effective. DDT powder is dusted on the clothes and body of the infested person. Clothes should be left for a while until all lice are dead, and then washed or cleaned. The patient should be bathed. In some countries, and under conditions of war, body lice have dangerous potentialities; they are known to be capable of spreading typhus, relapsing and trench fevers. As do head lice, body lice cause intense irritation and restlessness. Subsequent scratching may cause impetigo and swollen glands.

(3) The pubic louse—*phthirus pubis*—sometimes called the crab louse because of its shape, is similar in many ways to the head and body lice, but slightly smaller in size and nearly circular in outline. Crab lice are found in the axillary and pubic hair. Treatment is to shave the infested hair and treat the body and the clothes with DDT powder. Lice can be conveniently caught by using a piece of wet soap.

In all three cases infestation is due to direct contact with an infested person.

Sarcoptes scabei.—This is a tiny animal parasite which causes scabies. The mite gives rise to intense irritation, so the disease is often referred to as " the itch ". The insect tends to favour areas of the body where the skin is soft and delicate, as in between the fingers or on the front of the wrists. The male stays on the surface of the skin and the female burrows under the skin making tracks in which to lay about two dozen eggs. These take a few days to hatch and come out on to the surface where the females are fertilised by the male and start the process again. Intense irritation is caused which always seems much worse at night when the body is warm and the sarcoptes active. As a result of scratching with dirty nails impetigo may result.

Treatment, if properly carried out, is very effective. After a hot bath an emulsion of benzyl benzoate is applied over the whole body below the neck, especially over the infested areas. This is left to dry for about twenty minutes before the patient is allowed to dress. The patient takes a second bath after two days but should take care to apply a little of the emulsion *to his hands after washing*. Clothes should be *changed and washed*. It is important that other members of the family should also receive treatment, otherwise reinfestation will occur.

Bugs (cimex lectularius or bed bug).—These are parasites of reddish-brown colour, which live in the crevices and cracks of old walls, bedsteads and floors. They come out at night and suck the blood of humans, leaving a small red bite and causing irritation and restlessness. Eggs are laid in crevices and take eight days to hatch and about six weeks to mature into fully grown bugs. These bugs can live for as long as a year away from the human body. There is a peculiar smell in places infested with bed bugs.

Weapons of extermination against these bugs include strict cleanliness, hot water and soap, fresh air, sunlight and clean bed linen. The Local Authority will, if necessary, disinfest the building with DDT spray. DDT powder can be blown into all cracks and crevices. With old, badly infested buildings the only really successful measure is to rehouse the families after spraying furniture and goods, and to demolish the buildings.

Fleas (pulex irritans).—This is the flea that most commonly attacks man. It has a brown skin and can jump a considerable distance. Like the other parasites it lives by sucking blood. These fleas can be destroyed by ordinary cleanliness, plenty of hot water and soap, clean clothes, fresh air and sunlight. DDT powder can be sprinkled on to bedding and into cracks and crevices.

The Indian Rat Flea (xenopsylla cheopis).—This is a potentially dangerous parasite because it is capable of carrying plague. For this reason the Port Health Authorities exert careful control over ships coming into ports, particularly those carrying grain, to prevent possibly infested rats from coming ashore. Similarly on land, rats must be kept under control in all grain stores and warehouses, etc. The Rodent Officer of the Local Authority will deal with any infestation by rats if it is reported.

Ring-worm (Tinea).—There are several types of ring-worm, which results from a fungus infestation. The most relevant to this chapter is that affecting the scalp, called *Tinea capitis*. Dry scaly patches occur, and the hair breaks off. It is very contagious and is spread by infested hats, combs, hair brushes, etc. Diagnosis is confirmed by microscopic examination of the affected hairs or by means of a Woods glass screen and a mercury vapour lamp. The infestation may be of an animal or human kind.

In both kinds Whitfield's ointment may be rubbed into the lesions twice a day, but whereas the animal type usually succumbs to this treatment, the human type is more resistant. For the latter a single carefully regulated dose of X-ray may be necessary to make the infested hairs fall out. Whitfield's ointment is applied two days after epilation, and continued until the infestation is destroyed.

SEXUAL RELATIONS

Boys and girls reaching adolescence face challenges of healthy living in connection with their relations to the opposite sex. At this time it is important that activities occur which bring both sides together socially in healthy contact with each other. New drives which the adolescents feel need to be directed into healthy channels, and it is important for them to know the consequences of sexual relations outside marriage. By this time the normal reasonably adjusted boy or girl has learned to exercise self-discipline and restraint and should have knowledge of the dangers and symptoms of venereal disease.

The importance of parental influence cannot be over-estimated. Throughout the child's development their ability and willingness to give information clearly and directly as and when the child asks, or appears ready for it, is vital. The ability to respect and trust their children is important, but most influential of all is the natural love, concern and consideration shown by the parents for each other and for their children.

Heterosexuality is the term used to describe normal sexual relations between two people of opposite sex. The term Homosexuality refers to a less common relationship between two persons of the same sex. Close friendships with members of ones own sex occur as a normal part of the growing up process and some completely satis-factory heterosexual relationships may have been preceded by a degree of homosexual activity by one or other partner—but the man or woman who finds himself or herself quite unable to have sexual relationship with other than his or her own sex tends on the whole to be regarded by our present day society as abnormal and socially unacceptable, and persons who have strong tendencies in this direc-tion can suffer great isolation and feelings of guilt: others come to terms with their condition and form stable relationships with a partner of the same sex. A more sympathetic climate of opinion has grown up in recent years toward homosexual persons in the United Kingdom. Voluntary organisations exist to which they can turn for help, support and advice*.

Because of difficult customs this problem exists more in highly developed societies such as that of Great Britain and North America, but it does not seem to create the same concern in the less sophisticated countries. It is interesting to note that the incidence of syphilis among homosexuals is very high. In Great Britain no less than seventy per cent of early cases of syphilis are practising homosexuals.

Unnatural sexual relations between women is called Lesbianism and the law as it stands at present ignores this practice. Until 1970 in Great Britain the law forbad homosexual acts between males, but now has been amended to permit sexual acts between consenting males (over twenty-one years) providing these acts do not take place publicly and so do not constitute a public nuisance.

Although this is so there seems to be no definite provision for persons so affected. They do not as yet come under the umbrella of the National Health Services, but there can be no denying that they need help and understanding if they are to live healthy and happy lives.

PERSONAL HEALTH HAZARDS RELATED TO SOCIAL TRENDS

SEXUALLY TRANSMITTED DISEASES (STD)
VENEREAL DISEASE

The Venereal Diseases Act of 1917 which is still valid applies to syphillis, gonorrhoea, non-specific urethritis, soft chancre and other less serious diseases. The term "venereal" implies diseases transmitted by sexual intercourse and their control therefore presents social and medical problems in all countries and has done for many years. One might assume that as communities become more educated such diseases would be less prevalent but unfortunately this has not proved to be so. More than one disease may be suffered at one time by the same person.

There is little doubt that venereal disease is spread by sexual act, but fingers may be responsible for transferring the infection before the sexual act. Gonococcal vaginitis which occasionally occurs in children may be conveyed by contaminated fingers.

In the United Kingdom as in many European and North American

* Albany Trust, 32 Shaftesbury Avenue, London, W.1.

countries, there was a definite decline in incidence due to the discovery and effective use of Penicillin between the period 1940–1955 but this improvement was not maintained. Since 1955 many countries have experienced an alarming increase which may in part be due to increased population mobility and more widespread promiscuity.

Increased promiscuity may be the result of changing (or declining) moral standards. This increase should be a matter for concern to all who desire healthy living.

Since 1948 Regional Hospital Boards have had an obligatory responsibility for organising clinics—referred to as special clinics—in all areas. Everything is done to encourage those who have taken risks and those needing treatment to attend. Clinics for both sexes are open at convenient times and provision made to avoid publicity. Buildings and entrances are inconspicuous, there is no waiting and all evidence given is treated with strict confidence, but an amendment was made to the 1948 Act in December 1968 allowing information to be given to a doctor or special person employed by the doctor. This was done as a necessary measure to facilitate treatment and contact tracing in an attempt to control the increasing incidence of this disease. Venereal Diseases are not at present notifiable in the United Kingdom.

For overall control efforts are needed to raise moral standards by encouraging self control both in the use of alcohol and drugs, and in promiscuity.

Promiscuity means sexual intercourse with more than one partner and unrestricted by marriage: and statistics show that three-quarters of all venereal disease patients contract the disease whilst under the influence of alcohol.

A leading medical expert has said, "Moral standards are based upon stable family life and knowledge does not of itself bring virtue. Though our society may seem physically and mentally strong and healthy it is a matter for consideration whether its roots in family life may not be suffering from decay." These diseases are being transmitted by our young people—mainly the under twenty-fives. Educational programmes are being intensified—film*, television, newspapers and magazines are all vehicles for disseminating information.

The role of the general practitioner in controlling sexually transmitted diseases is important. Those practising in urban areas may have the assistance of a specially designated health visitor.

* 1963 " V.D. and Their Dangers " Available from the Central Film Library. 1970 "One Quarter of a Million Teenagers" Film obtainable from Boulton-Hawker Films Limited, Hadleigh, Suffolk.

The Public Health Committee of the Council of Europe gives advice and help to each member nation in the hope that the organisation of these services will be improved. Services must be established before control can be achieved in a situation where the movement of populations relating to tourism and migrant labour is already large and likely to increase. In countries with reliable notification systems, increase in sexually transmitted disease can be measured and compared. The main index is the case numbers per 100,000 of population for early syphilis and gonorrhoea.

Since 1972 the Joint Board of Clinical Nursing Studies has given attention to this need by developing post-basic training programmes for registered and enrolled nurses to enable them to work more effectively in special clinics. Because surveys showed that most of those currently employed in this work were of the older age groups younger students are encouraged. Intensive pilot schemes were centred in the large conurbations to help the DHSS to realise its intention to give all regions a well developed service particularly associated with district hospitals.

The number of clinics for sexually transmitted diseases that have been renamed departments of genito-urinary medicine has increased, without causing problems for doctors or patients.

Research projects are sponsored by the Medical Research Council, the DHSS and the World Health Organisation. In addition the World Health Assembly in 1975 passed a resolution highlighting the need to make optimum use of services, encourage the appropriate training of health personnel and health education to all concerned in order to develop the sense of responsibility and respect for the integrity of all human beings.

Venereal Disease Social Work. In the United Kingdom cities, especially seaports, a disproportionate amount of work is created by itinerant or socially unstable people. These people and their contacts are more difficult to trace and many will not complete treatment even when started.

The change in the law affecting male homosexuals makes it easier for men to discuss their problems and to seek treatment.

The advent of the Pill on the other hand has probably increased the incidence of venereal disease amongst young people by removing

Tables on pages 55 and 56. DHSS. On The State of Public Health 1973. Years 1971, 1972, 1973 reproduced by permission of the Controller, HMSO.

some of the fear of pregnancy resulting from premarital sexual relationships.

There is an urgent need to create more public awareness of the dangers of venereal disease and to make more factual information available.

The role of the S.T.D. Welfare Officer and social worker is largely concerned with contact tracing, and encouraging contacts to report for examinations and treatment. This officer is also instrumental in helping people who start treatment to complete it.

S.T.D. services have developed in the U.K. over the past half century but more particularly since 1948. The present plan is to ensure that all regions have an adequate service particularly associated with district general hospitals.

Syphilis. This disease has been known in Europe since the fifteenth century but it was not until early in the twentieth century that the causative organism was discovered. (1905, Schudin and Hoffman). It is a long thin thread wound in the form of a spiral and it is actively mobile. It is called the Treponema Pallidum, or the spirochaete of syphilis.

Syphilis tends to be more common in men than in women but can affect both. It is a most unpleasant disease and in its early stages it is inconspicuous and insidious and therefore often difficult to diagnose. It is highly infectious venereally and has a short incubation period—the usual is fourteen to twenty-eight days, but may have a range of nine to ninety days. The disease is diagnosed by serological blood tests but, in the past, tests available (Wassermann and Khan) have given rise to difficulties as both syphilis and yaws can give a positive result. Recently alternative and more reliable tests have been discovered. Regional Blood Transfusion Centres are responsible for doing routine serological tests on pregnant women and although the number of patients giving a positive result remains low, it is considered sufficiently significant to justify antenatal testing.

Syphilis is infectious in its early stages but not in what is called the late stage. Early syphilis comprises the primary, secondary, and early latent stages. Because of effective treatment late syphilis is declining but the disease has increased over the past twenty years. Much of the increase in early syphilis is found in male homosexuals between the age of 20–24 yrs. The ultimate results of this disease, untreated, are insanity, blindness and organic heart disease and it is when evidence of these conditions is seen that the term "Late" syphilis is appropriate. If a pregnant mother has syphilis the foetus may die in utero or be too badly diseased when born to survive long. If the baby does survive birth, disease can become evident later, affecting the ears by deafness, or the eyes by defective vision. In the past syphilis has been one of the main causes of blindness. It is for this reason that serological tests are made on all pregnant women as routine. Adequate treatment can be given which makes it possible for a diseased mother to have a healthy child.

Gonorrhoea. This disease is very old—so old that it is difficult to trace its origin. It was known in biblical times and is mentioned in connection with the early crusaders. The organism which causes it was first discovered and described in 1879 by Albert Neisser. It is called the Gonococcus and appears under magnification as a bean shaped organism which grows in pairs. Fifty per cent of female patients with Gonorrhoea are relatively asymptomatic. These cases are brought to the clinic by social workers as contacts of known male cases. All patients with Gonorrhoea can be cured.

Gonorrhoea is much more common than syphilis. It is equally unpleasant and is confirmed by taking a wet swab of the discharge and culturing the organism. It has a short incubation period—the usual is three to ten days but from twenty-four hours to twenty-one days is possible and early treatment with modern drugs is successful. Unfortunately many young girls who get infected live promiscuously and so become reinfected and the remedy therefore is rather more sociological than medical. This disease affects both sexes by causing acute inflammation of the lining of the reproductive tract with a subsequent purulent discharge. This is more easily noticed and detected in men but either sex can recognise when something is wrong—inflammation is painful and the discharge evident. In addition to this, toxins produced by the inflammation may affect delicate body tissues, for example the lining of the heart—endocardium, causing endocarditis, and the linings of the joints—synovia, causing synovitis (arthritis): in the eye, of the iris causing iritis: the urogenital tract in the male causing prostatitis and epididymitis and of the female causing salpingitis. An infected mother may be responsible for an infant developing an acute inflammation of the conjunctiva of the eyes, which get infected during the passage of the baby along the birth canal. This is called Ophthalmia Neonatorum. It is much less common than previously and is a notifiable disease.

It is to be regretted that like syphilis, the incidence of Gonorrhoea in Great Britain has risen steadily since the war and the rising numbers of young people requiring treatment gives cause for concern. Females tend to be less inclined to seek treatment because the early symptoms of gonorrhoea in the female are less unpleasant than in the male.

Non-gonococcal urethritis in males has been reported in a separate category since 1951 since when it seems also to have shown a steady increase. Women who contract this disease from male contacts are regarded as being on the increase. All patients with gonorrhoea can be cured.

SMOKING

In recent years three important reports,*†‡ have brought to the attention of the public, particularly to those responsible for the well-being of young people, dangers associated with smoking. Hospital authorities have been asked to give guidance and to review the existing rules on smoking in their own hospitals. The importance of the example set by staff—especially professional staff—is manifest. It is important to persuade young people, boys particularly, not to acquire the habit. The Children and Young Persons Act, 1963, increased by tenfold the penalties for selling tobacco to persons apparently under the age of sixteen, and the government has urged local authorities to set up anti-smoking clinics for those who wish to stop, but who have been unfortunate enough to develop the habit. Publicity material, posters§, films‖, and publicity vans are available. Social surveys are being carried out to assess the effect of the campaign and provide information to assist its development in future years. In January 1971 The Royal College of Physicians sponsored a new organisation "Action on Smoking and Health" (A.S.H.). This organisation called for a ban on smoking in places of entertainment and public transport. In August 1971 and again in 1977 Her Majesty's Government mounted an even greater campaign and provided funds for anti-smoking programmes on television.

Young people start smoking for various reasons, some of which are curiosity—just to see what it is like—a desire to be socially accepted —to do what others do—and a desire to behave in a grown-up way —to do what parents or admired adults do. Many of those who start in this way give up fairly quickly without ever acquiring the habit,

* Royal College of Physicians. United Kingdom, 1962.
† United States Public Health Service, 1964.
‡ Royal College of Physicians. Smoking and Health Now, 1971.
§ Obtainable from the Central Council for Health Education.
‖ Smoking and You. Obtainable from the Central Film Library, London W.3.

while others may become moderate or heavy smokers. Among those belonging to the latter group are those who smoke to pass the time away because they are committed for life to a dull and dreary job, or because tensions created by living require dampening down by some form of tranquillizer and smoking seems to be one of the least harmful. Some claim that smoking reduces a voracious appetite and so controls weight increase. Those who need to justify the smoking habit will use one or all of these arguments. For those of any age needing to be convinced, a study of tobacco and its constituents is a worthwhile exercise. Tobacco is made by fermenting and drying the leaf of the plant, and its chief component is a drug called nicotine; this is a volatile alkaloid (a colourless oily compound) and one of the most violent poisons known. The amount of nicotine in tobacco smoke varies not only with the kind of tobacco but with its dryness and the form in which it is burned. The amount that is absorbed by the body is influenced to some degree by the extent to which the smoke is inhaled. Because cigar and pipe smokers are less inclined to inhale they are considered to be less exposed to danger. In addition to nicotine there are other irritating substances in tobacco smoke, such as tar and carbon monoxide.

Tobacco is a narcotic, although its first effect upon the nervous system is stimulating. The first use of tobacco is usually accompanied by symptoms of poisoning—nausea, dizziness and headache —but smokers soon develop tolerance through use. Smokers with sedentary habits suffer heart and nerve effects more severely than those more active. People inclined to nervousness easily develop the smoking habit and soon find themselves unable to resist it for long. The effect upon mental activity varies; in some it calms the nerves while in others it produces headache and nervous irritability. It is known too that certain physiological changes are caused, such as increase in pulse rate and blood pressure, with a lowering of the temperature in the fingers and toes. There is also a loss of appetite usually accompanied by a loss in weight.

Prolonged excessive smoking sometimes produces disturbances in the loco-motor system of the body, manifested by fine tremor of the hands, clumsy movements with diminishing manual dexterity and deterioration in visual acuity. In addition, the delicate and important lining of the respiratory passages are chronically irritated and the individual becomes far more inclined to develop chest infections. Most important of all, statistics show a higher incidence of, and death rate from, lung cancer and coronary artery disease among heavy smokers than in other people. It is considered that cigarette smoking is now as important a cause of death as were the great epidemic diseases such as typhoid, cholera and tuberculosis. Research has also shown that mothers who smoke during pregnancy retard the growth of the unborn children. Particularly, this applies to the period after the third or fourth month of pregnancy. Babies born so affected may be described as "dismature", they are small and in addition have low blood sugar levels. The concentration of nicotine in the blood prevents glucose from getting to the brain cells which results in subsequent damage or retarded development. In addition to having smaller babies, they are more liable to lose their babies from abortion, still births and deaths in the first days of life. In addition there is evidence to suggest that they do not develop intellectually at the same rate as children born of non smoking parents. It is even suggested as a possible cause of mental subnormality.

One further fact to be considered is that smoking adds to the toll of accidental deaths. In Great Britain one hundred people a year die in fires annually, the cause of which were traced to smoking.

An intelligent understanding of these facts should help young people to resist this dangerous and useless habit. It is important to do so not only to protect them from its unfortunate consequences but also because if young people smoke heavily there is evidence to show that growth may be retarded, athletic performance affected and muscular power decreased with permanent fatigue. It is obvious that those who suffer from asthma or any respiratory disability should be warned emphatically against smoking.

Like all habits, smoking once established is hard to stop. It is relatively easier not to acquire the habit than to stop it once established. To resist the habit requires the understanding gained through education and the exercise of self-discipline. To stop the habit also requires self-discipline but in addition the substitution of better and less harmful ways of reducing nervous tension. An interesting occupation and relaxing and absorbing hobbies are good investments against starting this habit and can be equally effective in stopping it. If you are an established smoker and cannot or do not want to stop you should not use unfair persuasion to break other people's determination. To diminish the effect of smoking, try to reduce the amount of smoke inhaled, use filtered cigarettes and do not smoke the cigarette to the very end. Consider switching to pipe smoking or reduce the number you smoke each day by increasing the intervals between them. Better still, consider seriously trying to give it up altogether, and spend the money on something more useful, interesting and less harmful. A little time spent on simple arithmetic to show how much ten cigarettes a day for forty years will cost, may provide sufficient stimulus to save the money for something more constructive. It would probably go a long way toward providing the family with a house. Decide never to start or if you have started decide upon a special day when you will stop and make yourself keep to your decision.

Most important of all, as you grow older do not underestimate the importance of example set by you to the young you are privileged and bound to influence.

ALCOHOL AND ALCOHOLISM

Alcohol is produced by the fermenting of sugar with yeast. Grain and fruits are used in various ways to provide many different flavours. Alcohol affects the body physiologically by narcotic action although initially it appears to be stimulating. The exhilarating or stimulating effect of a mild or short drink is brought about by depression of the higher nerve centres that exercise inhibition so that the individual loses his usual social restraints. It has been said that behaviour begins to deteriorate as soon as there is any alcohol at all in the blood.

To some extent alcohol can be regarded as a food providing fuel for bodily combustion but apart from giving comfort to the elderly it is rarely justified medicinally, for there are cheaper and less harmful supplies of fuel available. Before anaesthetics were discovered alcohol was used in large amounts to produce sleep or complete stupor, and until recently, in small doses as an emergency stimulant. Anaesthetics and safer forms of stimulant are available now, and alcohol has become—in most developed communities— a social luxury and an easy source of revenue. Unfortunately it has become the root of a world-wide problem too because it is often taken in excess. The misuse of alcohol presents a far greater social problem than does the misuse of drugs. W.H.O. claims that alcoholism is the world's third major disease and is twenty times more prevalent than all other addictions combined. " Alcoholism " causes deterioration in personal health and damage to community life: and the revenue collected from those who drink alcohol could almost be offset by the national cost of unemployment, disease, poverty, delinquency, family welfare and accidental death or injury resulting from overindulgence. Alcohol produces severe dependence in 1 in 15 of all drinkers. Alcoholics occupy about 7,500 mental hospital beds, and they form a fair proportion of those who are homeless or who use reception centres. In Britain alone there are about 350,000–500,000 alcoholics* and absenteeism from work costs British industry at least £100 million a year.

The Misuse of Alcohol. Drunkenness, Alcoholic Intoxication and Alcoholism. Alcoholism is a complex condition described by many as a social disease characterised by the individual's inability to adapt himself to his environment without resource to excessive amounts of alcohol. There is no one single cause: it seems to be an expression of character and social attitude. The results however are indisputable. The sufferer and his family become a public health problem and a community responsibility. The alcoholic not only suffers varying degrees of economic decline, degradation and physical illness, and faces the possibility of insanity and death but also runs the risk of damaging the health and happiness of his (or her) family.

Alcoholism must be distinguished from alcoholic intoxication and drunkenness. The latter is betrayed by the external show of behaviour resulting from the action of alcohol on the brain cells. The uncontrolled, often noisy behaviour of any drunken person is unpleasant and undesirable and can lead to serious consequences for others as well as for himself. Drunkenness causing lessening of self control may lead to sexual misconduct, assault, hooliganism with wanton damage to property and cruelty to children and animals. No one who takes too much alcohol can be fit to work or to take responsibility. Recent reports published in the United Kingdom suggest that twenty per cent of fatal traffic accidents are considered to be due to misuse of alcohol. In the campaign for safety on the roads the following slogan is used " If you drive—don't drink and if you drink, don't drive." People are advised not to ride in a car that is being driven by someone who has been drinking. By doing so they put their safety in the hands of someone who is not fully responsible.†

Alcoholic intoxication can be described as a temporary state in which the level of alcohol in the blood is sufficient for the person

---

* Approximately one third of all alcoholics in Britain are women.

† The Road Safety Act 1962 made it an offence to drive if " a persons ability to drive properly is for the time being impaired ". This Act is still in force. The 1967 Road Traffic Act made it an offence to drive with a blood alcohol level higher than 50 mg/100 mh of blood.

Proof of impairment is enough to obtain a conviction even if the blood level is substantially below 80 mg/100 ml.

to be seriously affected. It must be remembered that this level varies in individuals according to their tolerance levels.

A percentage of those who habitually get drunk or suffer bouts of alcoholic intoxication will progress to become alcoholic addicts. Once this state has been reached the individual is a sick person. The alcoholic drinks not because he likes the taste or the feeling of pleasure that results, but because he must. The alcohol appears to help the individual to cope with his problems, but in fact, it merely helps him to forget them temporarily. It can be said that if you drink to drown your troubles you simply teach them to swim.

Of the many accepted definitions of the alcoholic, M. Mann's is brief but apt—" A person who drinks when he should not and must not, and wished he would not." (To substitute " need " for " would " seems to be even 'more appropriate.)   " Alcoholics are excessive drinkers whose dependence on alcohol is sufficient to affect their bodily and mental health, to damage their personal relations, and to degrade their social and economic status. They need treatment as soon as their conduct shows evidence of such results." (This is my own definition.)

The people most likely to be affected by alcohol in this way are those with certain psychological characteristics—they are inclined to be tense, with feelings of inadequacy and difficulties in the establishment of personal relationships. Technically they are said to be emotionally insecure. Alcohol removes, temporarily, inhibitions which ought not to be there. When the effects of the alcohol wear off the inhibitions return. Their temporary absence makes the drinker feel more secure, more integrated socially, more like a man: indeed he feels as he should feel if he were well adjusted, socially balanced: but it is a knife-edge kind of balance which few can maintain—it needs just what the drinker does not have, a sense of proportion. Unless he can reject alcohol as a permanent cure for his social difficulties he almost inevitably goes too far.

Once fully addicted to alcohol the individual gets an impulsive craving which if not indulged may lead to withdrawal symptoms such as delirium tremens, and convulsive fits. Because of associated anorexia complications are often due to malnutrition and vitamin deficiency.

To live normally the alcoholic must learn to cope with his difficulties in a more mature and less harmful way. He must find a balance in life without resorting to any chemical crutches. He can rarely—if ever—achieve the ability to enjoy ordinary social drinking without having a relapse. The alcoholic must give up alcohol completely, there can be no half measures for relapses will occur if alcohol is taken.

All members of the community should be aware of this and should try to understand the problem. They can help by remembering to provide non-alcoholic drink when arranging parties and by avoiding persuasion when someone has declined an offer of alcoholic liquor. Everyone has the responsibility of protecting himself and others from unhappiness.

The misuse of alcohol is becoming a serious world problem. In the United Kingdom where the disease is not as serious as in some other western countries, it has been suggested that alcoholism should be made a notifiable disease. For some years legislation was under consideration for laying down standard alcoholic tests for people suspected of being drunk in charge of cars. Five tests are possible for estimating the level of alcohol in the body—tests on the cerebro-spinal fluid, saliva, blood, urine and the breath. The "breathalizer" test has special advantages and in 1968 legislation was passed to legalise this test for strengthening the charge against any person suspected of being drunk in charge of a car. Unfortunately, some have already found ways of weakening the strength of this test. It is rapid, relatively simple, inexpensive and arouses little resistance. One controversial point seems to be that the level of tolerance varies in individuals. The then Minister of Health recommended the setting up of regional hospital units in psychiatric hospitals and psychiatric units in general hospitals, for the treatment of alcoholism: and intending nurses and social workers were encouraged to equip themselves by study to help with the problem.

Although the United Kingdom is not yet facing such a serious problem as are some other countries it is indeed serious enough and we should not be complacent but do everything we can to protect our young people and to help those already afflicted.

Recently a memorandum to local health authorites drew attention to the need for statutory and voluntary services to work together, to provide a comprehensive service for prevention, assessment, treatment and aftercare. In addition the Standing Mental Advisory Committee having reviewed existing arrangements, have asked Regional Health Authorities to extend the provision of special treatment centres to those regions where they did not previously exist.

"Alcoholics Anonymous " and other existing organisations.
Alcoholics Anonymous is an association or fellowship created by and

wholly composed of alcoholics who have found recovery or are still seeking it. They consider alcoholism to be a disease and the alcoholic a sick person. Started in 1935 it is now well established in the United States and Europe and will help anyone who wishes to be cured. Alcoholics Anonymous supplements medical treatment and the prognosis depends on the patients' attitude to change. Recovery rates vary; they are very favourable among those who co-operate fully.

In addition to this association many large cities in the United Kingdom have Alcoholics Information Centres and some psychiatric and general hospitals now accept sufferers as out-patients for diagnosis and treatment.

A telephone call to A.A. will bring prompt help or information. In most cities and towns there is a local A.A. office. A.A. aims to work in co-operation with the professional and all other sections of the community. All contribute to the total circle of help needed around the alcoholic.

The Professional Relations Committee of the A.A. has recently set up a new committee called the General Service Board. Its objectives are to bring about more communication, understanding, respect and cooperation between Alcoholics Anonymous and any professional person who works with alcoholics.

DRUG ADDICTION OR DEPENDENCE

Drug addiction is a world-wide problem; it is not a new one, but has undoubtedly become more widespread since easy means of travelling have become available to the " man in the street ". During the twentieth century, and particularly since the second world war, it has aroused increasing attention because younger people have become affected. Organisations like the United Nations provide channels for information, international discussion and co-operation.

Although the " black-spots " are to be found in big cities and sea-ports, drug addiction respects neither race, religion, neighbourhood nor economic status. No area or community is free from its dangers. The countries of the East, e.g. Burma, Hong Kong, Shanghai, Japan, China and Middle East countries such as Egypt, Syria, Palestine provide the more dangerous drugs. Cuba and Mexico also provide some which probably find their way into the neighbouring United States of America.

Most dangerous drugs are obtained from plants. The crude drugs are extracted and purified, either in the country of origin or in the receiving country. The most serious drugs that we are concerned with are opium, morphine, heroin, cocaine and cannabis.

Unfortunately master smugglers seldom carry drugs themselves. Male and female agents are used who do not know the names of the organisers or will not disclose them. Members of ships crews are obvious agents who use all kinds of devices to distribute the drugs in their crude or prepared states. They have even been known to make use of their special knowledge of ship construction for the purpose of avoiding detection: they shift the drugs from one part of the ship to another whilst officials are searching for it. False-bottomed suitcases, trunks, hollow-soled shoes, hollow heels, concealed pockets in clothing and even body orifices and cavities have been used.

When the agent has safely handed over his consignment of drugs, distribution is easy in countries with good communications. The drugs pass eventually to " sellers " or " pushers " who may first give them to possible victims as bait. When the victims have taken enough to want more they must buy it. Drugs are expensive and to find enough money addicts often resort to crime. The drugs affect them morally and socially and they often lose their jobs.

The term "habit" used to be distinguished from "addiction". A habit-forming drug was considered to be one which produced physical dependence, and there are many of them, but they do not cause withdrawal symptoms, neither do they affect the patient morally. Addiction, on the other hand, was considered to cause general deterioration in both physical and moral health, producing psychological dependency and withdrawal symptoms. Addiction was defined as " A condition in which a person compulsively misuses a drug to such an extent that both his health and his contribution to society deteriorate."

The causes of addiction are difficult to pinpoint, but it is most likely to affect those of weak character; the maladjusted, irresponsible, selfish, immature or thrill-seeking individuals. Initial contact with the addictive drug is of course necessary. People who suffer from chronic disease can become addicted to drugs prescribed for them but if they do, there is usually some contributory maladjustment. Some patients in the terminal stages of painful diseases become addicted, but they receive their drugs under medical supervision and do not constitute a threat to society.

Many addicts begin taking drugs before the age of twenty; and many persons start using drugs without realising how difficult it will be to stop and without understanding the serious consequences.

Marihuana cigarettes are a potential danger in that they offer a first step to addiction. Marihuana is a drug of habit rather than of addiction but does cause some slight psychological dependency, and therefore serves as a prelude to more sophisticated drugs.*

The organisation which exercises international control over illicit drugs, now centred at Geneva, seeks an increasing number of reports from governments of various countries. Using this information, it seeks the co-operation of governments of countries reported as the sources of drugs. The co-operation of seamen's unions is sought in an effort to reduce the number of seamen acting as carriers. Appeals to governments have been passed to their medical services, which have reduced the amount of heroin used medicinally. In some countries its legal use has been eliminated.

Dangerous Drugs Acts in force in most countries make it a legal obligation to keep all drugs of addiction under lock and key, and allow only qualified persons to obtain and administer them. Controllers of medical institutions, doctors, dentists, pharmacists and veterinary surgeons, must abide by these regulations, which attempt to prevent drugs required for medical purposes from reaching the illicit market. Pharmacists must be on the lookout constantly for forged prescriptions. Medical practitioners are urged to prevent blank prescription sheets from getting into unprofessional hands.

Most people who have become addicted can be cured if they make the effort and want to be helped. Long and skilful psychiatric treatment is required and rehabilitation is most important. Discharged patients need the sympathetic understanding and help of friends and family, and the support of family doctors and employers in making real adjustment to the stresses of life instead of again resorting to drugs as a form of escape.

Nurses and doctors have a special responsibility for safeguarding the supplies of the drugs they use in their work: and of course for resisting, privately and collectively, the inevitable temptation to use them personally.

An Advisory Council on the Misuse of Drugs was brought into operation in January 1972 to advise the Home Secretary and the Minister concerned with Health and Education, on measures which ought to be taken to deal with the medical and social problems connected with the misuse of drugs.

The Department provides facilities, through the Regional Health Authorities, for the treatment of addicts. Every encouragement is

* Note. A booklet "Drug Dependence" first published in June 1967—Wood. Available from Bristol Health Department.

given to voluntary organisations to provide hostels of various kinds, day centres, counselling and information services. Health education is emphasised in addition to developing improved links and communication between voluntary organisations, local authority and other statutory agencies. In 1972 financial assistance was given to Standing Conference on Drug Abuse (SCODA) with these aims in mind.

Addicts receiving narcotic drugs at 31st December
United Kingdom 1969–73.

	1969	1970	1971	1972	1973
No. of addicts	1,466	1,430	1,555	1,619	1,818

Also

Age, sex and treatment characteristics of addicts known to be receiving treatment at 31st December 1971.

Age	Methadone			Heroin			Other narcotic drugs			Grand total
	M	F	T	M	F	T	M	F	T	
Under 20	76	26	102	9	0	9	4	3	7	118
20–34	785	190	975	90	24	114	24	10	34	1,123
35–49	34	15	49	15	9	24	21	18	39	112
50 or over	14	12	26	5	4	9	46	98	144	179
Not known	5	4	9	—	—	—	7	7	14	23
	914	247	1,161	119	37	156	102	136	238	1,555

Reproduced by permission of the Controller, HMSO, from *On the State of the Public Health 1972*, and *1973*

THE BATTERED BABY SYNDROME

The term battered baby or battered child† syndrome is used to describe a clinical condition which results from serious physical or mental maltreatment of young children by their parents or other adults.

† Non Accidental Injury or Child Abuse or Concealed Parental Violence are alternative terms.

Since 1946 there has been a steadily increasing interest in and attention to this condition. This may be because the incidence has actually increased or merely because the increased attention has led to more frequent diagnosis. Boys tend to be the subjects more often than girls and premature babies more often than others.

Many adults who injure children have long standing emotional problems which might be remediable, and their behaviour might be a cry for help. Such adults may come from any social class. They are often described as psychopathic (mentally sick) or sociopathic (socially sick) characters. They sometimes indulge in alcohol and promiscuous sexual relationships. They tend to make unsuitable marriages and to commit minor crimes. They are often immature, impulsive, self-centred, over sensitive, quick to react and unable to control their aggression, which is expressed in physical violence. However, it also occurs in those with good education and stable financial and social backgrounds, but sometimes there is a suggestion that such people might themselves have suffered similar abuse in childhood, or been subject to rejection, indifference or hostility from their own parents or guardians.*

One must not forget that young parents even when quite normal have problems with babies and young children and if over-whelmed by stress and sleepless nights, might temporarily lose control.

Early recognition is important and attention should be alerted when a baby or young child is seen with a fracture of a bone, subdural hoematoma (head injury), failure to thrive, soft tissue swelling, skin bruising, repeated injuries or in the event of the sudden death of a young child. Suspicion is aroused when the degree and type of injury is at variance with the history.

Preventive measures are important if a repetition of the maltreatment on the same child or other siblings is to be avoided. Especially is it important to realise that protective and supportive help given by all kinds of professional workers to potential child abusers might be the most important element in prevention. There is a need for all who work with children to share information and work together; to develop efficient methods of speedy relay and accurate recording of messages. Effective and timely communication between schools, housing departments, police, the community, the N.S.P.C.C. and social services may prevent a child being harmed.

Some Area Review Committees to co-ordinate the agencies concerned are in operation and more will be established.

---

* The battered baby of today becomes the baby batterer of tomorrow.

HYPOTHERMIA

Cold can kill; it is vital to keep warm in winter. Everyone should be made aware that health is affected and life at risk when the body temperature drops well below the normal range—below 35° C (95° F) (rectal)*. The very young and the elderly are most at risk in countries whose climate includes spells of very cold weather.

All members of staff in National Health and Social Service departments should be aware of the dangers of this condition and alert to the signs, so that appropriate action may be taken to save life.

Preventive action offers the main hope of success but is difficult to implement. The very young and old exposed to cold and possibly undernourished, are the most likely sufferers, so that all schemes which involve the statutary and voluntary services in the provision of food and warmth to the needy should be encouraged.

Hypothermia as Applied to Babies

Normal babies as well as those prematurely born are incapable of regulating their temperature; especially is this so during the first three months of life. For this reason baby clothes and cot coverings should be light weight and warm and the air temperature in the room adequate. The cot needs protection from draughty doors and windows and the room made warmer when the baby is undressed for bathing (21° C—70° F—at least).

If the baby is found cold—the face and extremities are good indices—the doctor, midwife or health visitor should be called immediately and the room temperature raised as quickly as possible. It is important to avoid hot water bottles or extra heavy or tight clothing. The former can be dangerous if placed in contact with the baby and heavy tight clothing will restrict the baby's movements.

Young babies should never be left alone in the house, and those left responsible should know where to get help, if needed.

Hypothermia as Applied to the Elderly

The elderly person is less active and therefore more vulnerable to the cold. It is most important to see that the elderly are properly fed and have at least one warm room to live in. A temperature about 18° C (65° F) is preferable and one below 10° C (50° F) is dangerous.

Damp and heat loss should be prevented, but in so doing it is important to ensure adequate ventilation and safety with heating appliances.

* Special low reading thermometers are available.

In the absence of family or friends willing or able to help an elderly person who cannot afford room modifications or extra heating appliances, voluntary or local authority social service funds may be available.

If found in a state of hypothermia the aim of treatment is the natural and gradual restoration of body temperature to normal. This can be achieved by warming the whole room, giving the person a warm drink and providing extra warm, light-weight clothing and bed covers—hot water bottles can be dangerous and are best avoided.

Clearly it is important to visit old people during cold spells and to advise the doctor or health visitor of situations which cause concern.

CARE OF THE DYING. TERMINAL CARE

As communities become more developed—Westernised—preventive medicine more effective, the expectation of life rises. While it is recognised that many deaths follow brief and acute illnesses, it is also realised that a large number of patients reach a stage where curative treatment has nothing more to offer. Provision is therefore necessary for varying periods of terminal care.

Our habits of modern living have created and continue to exacerbate the problem. There is less spare room in the modern dwelling; the family budgeting is often geared to both partners working; and families are often living apart and the spouse, if still alive, is unable to carry such a burden. For these various reasons the family is less often than in the past, able to provide the care that is needed even with the provision of extended social services.

If given a choice, most people prefer to die in their own home near or with members of their own family. General medical, domiciliary nursing and personal social services are all geared to give supportive help but the strain on the family is never-the-less heavy.

The number of deaths occurring each year remains fairly constant —the greater proportion die in hospital but better, more suitable, provision is needed. It is often difficult to obtain a bed, the bed when obtained is not always in the best place, and nursing provision is insufficient. Dying patients need gentle and unhurried care and to many it seems inappropriate, psychologically and economically, to nurse such patients in acute wards.

In 1972 a National Symposium was held to which over 50 organisations were able to contribute. It is hoped that their deliberations will help toward wider knowledge and better understanding upon which an effort to strengthen the support we give, and the provision we make, can be based.

This is one of the challenges facing the newly formed Regional Health Authorities and to which Health Care Planning Teams will need to give attention.

It is estimated that of 7.5 million people in Great Britain over 65 yrs over a third of a million are in old peoples homes or in hospitals. At least a quarter of a million require domiciliary care.

PETS AND DISEASES

Pets provide fun and affection for children in addition to comfort and company for many elderly and otherwise lonely people. It must, however, be remembered that there are diseases, some serious, that can be transmitted by pets. Zoonosis is the collective name for these. Children are more vulnerable than adults but if common sense rules are obeyed the risks are slight.

Pets' boxes, cages and bedding should be kept clean; the latter washed regularly or safely destroyed. Food dishes kept clean and washed separately and animals prevented from licking household crockery. Pets need to be fed regularly on wholesome food and not allowed to lick food intended for humans.

Animals need regular grooming and the vet consulted if the pet appears sick. Excreta or vomit should be buried or burned and the animal taught to avoid soiling paths, play areas and lawns. Domestic food should be protected at all times and careful attention given to hand-washing after handling animals and before preparing or handling food.

It is most important to keep pets, especially dogs, properly controlled so that they do not constitute a nuisance or danger to others. Certain laws of the land are made to safeguard animals as well as individuals.

THE HEALTH EDUCATION SERVICE

The D.H.S.S. has an important role in promoting health education as a vital part of preventive medicine.

The Secretary of State delegates his national responsibility to a Health Education Council. The Council in turn delegates operational responsibility to the Area Health Authorities. To decide on the nature of campaigns and enable the Council to advise the area teams, a research committee, serviced by professional and administrative officers meets regularly. This committee reviews research findings, identifies fields of activity and makes recommendations regarding the financing of appropriate research. Decisions must also be made as to which are the most suitable agencies to undertake particular research projects.

This committee, in conjunction with the Health Education Council organises and conducts mass media campaigns, such as those directed against smoking and advocating the need for family planning.

The area teams are directed by a health education officer who has the assistance of other professional workers. Technical and secretarial staff are also employed to give support. The teams make themselves available to the community and are able to supply a wide range of materials for the purpose of influencing opinion. Group therapy sessions can provide a valuable contribution to their work. They also organise in-service education and training sessions for national health service staff working in primary and secondary schools.

SECTION III

DOMICILIARY AND COMMUNAL HEALTH

FOOD

Care of Food and Milk in the Home and Hospital—Food Hygiene Regulations. Many diseases may be spread by unwholesome food. Before considering these in detail, we must first describe the regulations designed to improve the care of food in order to reduce the risk of spreading disease.

The Sale of Food and Drugs Amendment Act of 1879 was the first to require local authorities to appoint public analysts to examine samples of food. Since then Section 13 of the Food and Drugs Act has been repealed and a number of new provisions made by the Food Hygiene Regulations 1955, which came into force in January 1956.

The regulations lay down requirements in respect of:

(1) The cleanliness of food premises and stalls, etc., and of apparatus and equipment.

(2) The hygienic handling of food.

(3) The cleanliness of persons engaged in the handling of food, and of their clothing, and the action to be taken where they suffer from, or are carriers of, certain infections.

(4) The construction of food premises, the repair and maintenance of such premises, stalls, vehicles, etc., and the facilities to be provided.

(5) The temperature at which certain foods liable to transmit disease are to be kept in food premises.

The new and wide definition of " food business ", which includes schools, clubs and works canteens, institutions, etc., removes any doubt as to the extent of legislative control over such premises, and also brings boarding houses and private hotels under control.

The tendency to belittle the value of food hygiene is not so evident as it was in years gone by; indeed, strong public opinion on all sides now supports the Health Authorities' reasonable requirements.

This careful control exercised by Health Authorities is fortified by work of an educational character, to make sure that people handling food in food stores, canteens, restaurants and in the home will perform, as a habit, those precautions dictated by common sense and common decency. This Clean Food Campaign combined with routine inspections should bring about an overall improvement and a lessening of outbreaks of food poisoning.

Although in the last few years there has been a fair amount of control, and epidemics of serious diseases spread by food have been reduced, the number of outbreaks of food poisoning especially in schools and hospitals still causes concern. It is reported that there are now from ten to fifteen more outbreaks of food poisoning per annum than before the war.

Whether food is stored, bought and prepared in the home, restaurant or hospital, many points apply, and for an intelligent understanding of the problem it is well to consider the following:

(1) *Selective Purchasing.*—Young people should be taught by their parents and school how to recognise food that is fresh, particularly when it is fish or meat. They should buy only from shops whose owners take the trouble to keep themselves and their premises clean, and the food covered and properly wrapped. Licking fingers and blowing into paper bags, together with unnecessary exposure and handling of food is to be condemned. Animals of all sorts should be under control and food protected from flies and dust. If everyone insisted on such a standard, shop-owners would have to conform or close down.

(2) *A high standard of hygiene in personal habits for those responsible for handling food.* This applies to everyone. Children should be taught to wash their hands after going to the lavatory and before sitting down to a meal, to use clean utensils rather than fingers— adults should set a good example. All persons having the responsibility of preparing or serving food should be free from infections, particularly those affecting the alimentary and respiratory systems. Any cuts or lesions of the fingers should be protected with waterproof covers. Clean, well-cut finger nails, clean aprons and suitable cover for the hair should be insisted upon for those working in communal kitchens. Proper toilet facilities should be provided near at hand and adequate arrangements for washing hands.

Bread and butter, if cut on a machine, should be transported in clean closed containers, and all foods such as cakes, or bread and butter, handled with clean food tongs, not with fingers. Food containers in hospitals, schools, hotels and restaurants should be transported properly covered on special food trolleys and not carried in or under the arms of porters or maids. Personnel handling food in the kitchens or serving food of any sort should be sufficiently intelligent to be taught the dangers of carelessness, shown simple films illustrating the right and wrong ways to handle crockery, utensils, etc., the care of their hands and persons, and given every encouragement to wear clean overalls. Smoking while working in the kitchen and serving food should be condemned.

(3) *Extermination and Control of Rodents, Flies and Insects of all sorts.*—All forms of breeding grounds, such as exposed rubbish dumps, uncovered bins, uncared for lavatories, dust and dirt of any sort should be eliminated. All food should be kept covered and as cool as possible—ideally in the household refrigerator. A cool store cupboard with a ventilated fly-proof door is the next best thing. Bread should be in a bin, safe from mice; and food not left exposed on the table; such things as sugar, jam, milk, cheese, butter, meat and fish serve as great attractions for flies and can easily be contaminated by them. Milk is best left covered in the bottle in which it is supplied until it is required for use. In hot weather the bottle can be stood in cold water.

(4) *Cooking and Food Storage.*—Before being cooked all food should be washed clean with reliable water and handled as little as possible; then bearing in mind that it still may be infected it should be heated quickly. After adequate cooking, if not used at once it should be cooled rapidly, and then placed in a reliable store cupboard or refrigerator. No food should be left to stand in a warm kitchen; this applies particularly to custards and gravy which are best made immediately before being required. Dried egg mixtures and milk powders should be used immediately after being reconstituted, and not allowed to stand in a warm room. Duck eggs and dried and frozen egg mixtures need very thorough cooking. Food which has been previously cooked and stored should be thoroughly heated before being eaten, not just warmed—this particularly applies to meat pies and gravy. Canned foods of any sort should be eaten as soon as opened, and frozen foods not kept after being removed from the deep freeze. Any tin that is misshapen and " blown " should be discarded, so also should fermented bottled fruit. Cooking utensils should be kept clean and in good repair, for minute quantities of metal, copper, zinc or lead from damaged utensils have, from time to time, caused poisoning.

(5) *The Kitchen Itself.*—Much thought and planning has gone into the design of modern kitchens, and given such design the care is relatively easy; but many hotels, schools, restaurants, hospitals and houses have to function with grossly inadequate arrangements.

The walls, ceiling and floors should be kept clean, so also should cupboard tops, sinks and draining boards. The latter are preferably made of stainless steel, porcelain or plastic material—the old type of wooden sink and board should be condemned. There should be adequate arrangements for the discharge of used water and a supply of reliable water. Hot water is a distinct advantage and may be provided by means of a heating unit above the sink, or some form of immersion heater, if a central boiler is not available. Provision should be made for the salvage of waste food. In cities and towns it may be collected regularly for pig swill—the container used must be kept clean and covered, and care taken not to put anything in it that would endanger the health of the pigs. Rubbish bins should not be kept in the kitchen. A good detergent and hot water is best used for washing up, care being taken not to use it too strong so that it damages the skin. The use of hot clean water for rinsing (used in conjunction with a draining board and plate rack) is an advantage. Dishcloths and mops should be kept clean, frequently boiled and regularly changed. Lighting should be adequate. Table tops of plain hardwood should be kept very clean, but many materials—enamel, Formica—are now being used most successfully to cover them. The latter is expensive but very pleasant to use, hardwearing and attractive. Ovens, saucepans, cooking utensils, should be kept clean and in good repair. All these things apply equally to small and large kitchens, but in the latter it is usual to have separate sink units for dealing with vegetables. For rinsing, very hot water is used, so that plates, etc., dry readily on draining racks, or alternatively, washing-machines may be used. It is usual in large kitchens to need some form of steam extractor, and in very large kitchens some form of artificial ventilator. Walls and floors are best tiled or made of a hard material which is easily washed. There should be adequate facilities for emptying water used for scrubbing the floors; it should not be tipped down the kitchen sink.

(6) *Notification of all Cases of Known or Suspected Food Poisoning, or Diseases Spread by Food.*—It is important for everyone to understand that by this notification further spread of the disease may be prevented. It gives the Community Physician a chance to ascertain the cause of poisoning or the source of infection. To enable him to do so, it is important to save any scraps of food that might reasonably have been responsible. These should be kept cool until removed for examination.

(7) *The Different Types of Food Poisoning*—how they are caused

and prevented, and diseases of the alimentary system that are spread by food will be dealt with later.

Control of Purity and Quality of Food. The control of purity and quality of food has advanced considerably since the Act of 1879. In those days substances were added to food for three main reasons: to improve its appearance as well as its keeping quality and to gain financially by adding cheap ingredients. The two former practices are known as " sophistication " and are allowed. The third, adulteration, is not. Heavy penalties are now imposed if adulteration of food is proved. As well as this, the offender would naturally suffer by losing a considerable amount of trust and consequently trade. Nowadays only a small percentage of samples of food taken are found to be adulterated or defective in quality. Only a limited number of preservatives are now allowed to be used, and these only in certain foods in stated proportions. The authorities are constantly aware of fresh problems, such as those arising from new methods of preserving food and from the use in horticulture of many new chemical fertilisers and pest-control sprays. A constant watch is kept on their effect on health and nutrient value. More recently attention is being directed to the effect of radio-active contamination of milk produced by cows fed on contaminated grass.

Certain Government departments, such as the Ministries of Health and that of Agriculture, Fisheries and Food, play an important part in supervising the quality and, incidentally, the quantity of certain food supplies. To help them they have the advice of the Food Hygiene Advisory Committee. As well, the Local Authority is responsible for taking samples of all kinds of food and drink. The Community Physician, the Public Analyst and the Health Inspector all have a part to play. A daily inspection of fish, fruit and vegetable markets is carried out, and a close watch kept on all food exhibited for sale, in shops, restaurants, on stalls or in travelling vans. The authority is concerned not only with the soundness of the food, but also with its nature, substance and quality. In one city of half a million population, 5,500 samples are submitted each year for bacterial and chemical analysis. Meat inspection is also very important—all carcasses and offal are examined, and any that do not satisfy the inspectors are condemned as unfit for human consumption.

Wholesale and retail premises, port buildings, abattoirs, factories and shops also are carefully inspected. Owners of unsatisfactory premises can be refused renewals of licences if they do not take steps to make the necessary improvements.

Regulations are in force relating to meat inspection, milk purity and designation, pasteurisation of liquid egg, bread, flour, and soft drinks.

The Ministry continues to have representatives on all committees and subcommittees concerned with the safety and composition of food.

Milk. *Control of the Purity and Quality of Milk. Designations of Milk.*—The authorities of this country realise that milk is probably one of the most valuable foods we possess. It is of vital importance to infants, young children, nursing and pregnant women. For this reason, during and between the last two world wars every effort was made to maintain the quality and improve the quantity of milk. Whilst appreciating its food value, one must realise also that it can be a serious source of danger because of the readiness with which organisms thrive in it.

The Minister of Health and Social Services and the Minister of Agriculture, Fisheries and Food jointly exercise powers to control the purity and quality of milk. The Central Government Authority plays an essential part in supervising its production by controlling registration of producers and their premises. The Local Authority supervises the distribution, but the consumer—particularly the housewife—also has an important part to play. Various schemes have been introduced as incentives to farmers to produce better and safer milk, and every form of encouragement used to persuade children and mothers to drink more.

Supervised by these authorities the control of purity is in the hands of:

(*a*) The farmer.

(*b*) The distributor.

(*c*) The consumer.

(*a*) *The farmer* is responsible for seeing that his cows are healthy. They must be free from obvious disease. A cow suffering from tuberculosis, undulant fever or streptococcal infection may give infected milk. This is particularly so if the cow has mastitis. The farmer also has the responsibility of seeing that his dairyman is fit to handle his cows. He must be free from infections of the upper respiratory tract, and the intestinal tract. Any lesions of the skin must be adequately covered. He must be of reliable hygienic habits, keeping his person and clothes clean, and washing his hands after going to the lavatory—adequate toilet facilities must be provided. The dairyman should be sufficiently intelligent to be aware of the dangers of carelessness.

Reliable water must be used for washing the flanks and udders of the cows, the milking utensils and the milker's hands, etc. Milking and cooling apparatus must be regularly inspected and cleaned, and the cow sheds and dairies kept clean and reasonably free from dung. They should be well constructed, properly lighted and ventilated and free from rodents and vermin. Domestic animals should be under control. It is also the farmer's responsibility to see that his milk is conveyed to the distributors in clean churns as soon after production as possible, from safe and suitable collecting places. Whilst awaiting collection churns should be protected from the heat of the sun. Large amounts may be conveyed in huge tanks to which it is passed by closed circuit directly from the cooling plant. Milk from the farm is known as *raw milk*. Laboratory tests on this show to what extent the farmer has been successful in producing pure milk.

(b) *The Distributor.*—The farmer may be the distributor also, or the milk from several farms may be pooled and dealt with by a distributing firm. Milk produced from a registered tuberculin attested herd need not undergo pasteurisation, but all other milk retailed to the general public must. Because of the human element most authorities consider it desirable to pasteurise all raw milk. If the milk is not received by the distributor in bottles it is first scrutinised and smelt by an expert, and frequent samples of the raw milk are taken to check composition as well as cleanliness. If accepted as wholesome, the milk is passed to the pasteurisation unit. This first filters the milk and then subjects it to rapid heat treatment, using a unit known as a heat exchanger. In this apparatus heat is transferred to the milk very rapidly through a pack of thin plates of stainless steel. In a few seconds a temperature of 72°C is reached and maintained for 15 seconds only, the milk is then rapidly cooled by abstraction of heat through a further set of stainless steel plates chilled by refrigeration. The rapidity of the process ensures that no damage is done to the milk, and at the same time absolute safety is achieved by the destruction of harmful organisms. On this machine there is automatic temperature and time recording, and a device which returns milk which has not been sufficiently heated.

This method of pasteurisation is known as the High Temperature, Short Time method (H.T.S.T.)—there are others but the speed of this one and the excellence of its results are tending to make it the most used.

After cooling, the milk is passed through a closed circuit to the automatic bottling plant. The empty bottles into which the milk

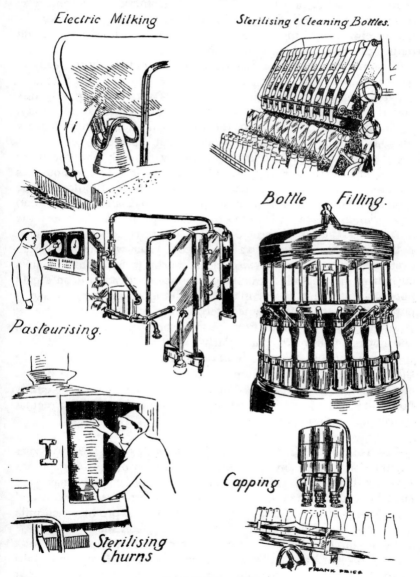

Fig. 23. The Story of Milk.

is poured have just left the automatic washing and sterilising machine, from which they are brought by a mechanical conveyer. The machinery immediately caps the sterilised bottles, covering the lips completely. The checked, filled, sealed bottles are then put into a refrigerating store until they can be distributed. Disposable wax cartons are being introduced to facilitate easier and quieter distribution of milk. Once the changeover has been completed they should reduce the cost of labour and equipment.

The milk churns are mechanically washed and sterilised, ready to be returned to the farm.

All the apparatus used in the processes above is regularly dismantled and cleaned, and tests are carried out to ensure reliability.

Finally, the distributor keeps the milk in cold storage until delivery time. If not sold it should be kept in a suitable place.

(c) *The Consumer.*—To maintain purity of milk, the consumer should ensure regular supplies, should take it into the house as soon as possible, and if it has to remain outside, should provide protection from sun and immunity from animals and birds. A cup or special cover can be inverted over the top. Inside the house the milk is best left in its sealed bottle in a refrigerator or ice box. Failing this, it can be stood in a bowl of cold water, with a cup inverted over the top and draped with clean muslin, where possible in a current of air. In cold weather it is sufficient to stand it on a cold floor or ledge in a cold cupboard. It is advisable not to take it out of the bottle until immediately before it is required for use. Jugs, etc., used for containing the milk should be absolutely clean, and not left uncovered, particularly in hot weather.

To guarantee the continuity of daily deliveries, it is necessary for the dairies to stock large numbers of spare bottles. These bottles are expensive; the housewife should play her part by washing empty bottles, rinsing them in cold water and putting them out for regular collection by the milkman.

Control of Quality. The quality of milk from healthy cows should not vary to any great extent, and according to regulations may not fall below certain standards. The fat content may vary slightly from summer to winter, and also with breed of cow and quality of pasture. Certain breeds are known to produce rich milk and also those fed in certain localities, e.g. Cornwall.

In Britain, cows' milk must contain not less than 3 per cent. milk fat and 8.5 per cent. milk solids other than fat. If the milk falls below this standard it is assumed to have been adulterated, or that the cows are producing poor milk—probably because of poor feeding. The latter is investigated by analysis of milk taken directly from the cows. If it is proven, efforts must be made by the farmer to improve the feeding. One test to find out if water has been added to milk is to test the freezing point—addition of water causes it to be raised.

DESIGNATIONS OF MILK

There are three main designations of milk now recognised:

(1) Tuberculin Tested (T.T.).

(2) Pasteurised.

(3) Sterilised.

(1) *Tuberculin Tested.*—This is milk obtained from cows especially registered as being healthy and free from tuberculous infection. The farmer who owns such a herd must have a special licence and conform to certain regulations. An effort is being made to encourage farmers to produce Tuberculin Tested milk; certain areas, called " Specified Areas " are selected as and when opportunities arise. Milk from these " specified areas " must be pasteurised if it is not from Tuberculin Tested cows. Farmers are paid a better price for this higher grade of milk and every encouragement is given in the Specified Areas to raise tuberculous-free herds. Tuberculin Tested milk may also be pasteurised (Tuberculin Tested Pasteurised). This makes it doubly safe and renders the milk absolutely free from any other form of infection. Tuberculin Tested milk may be sterilised (Tuberculin Tested Sterilised).

(2) *Pasteurised Milk*—is milk heated to a temperature between 63°C and 65°C for a period of thirty minutes, or to a temperature of 72°C or above for a period of at least 15 seconds, before being cooled to a temperature not exceeding 10°C.

The farmer may hold a licence to pasteurise milk on his farm, or send it to a pasteurising establishment. The bottles or other containers must be filled on the pasteurising premises.

(3) *Sterilised Milk.*—This is required to be filtered or clarified, homogenised and heated in bottles to a temperature not below 94°C, for such a period as will ensure that it complies with a prescribed test. Milk so treated is completely germ-free, but the taste is altered and the vitamin C destroyed.

" Raw " is the term used to describe milk straight from the cow, and not treated in any way. Only a small percentage of milk consumed in this country at present is " raw ".

If the farmer is sufficiently equipped to bottle his milk on the farm, then " farm bottled " may be added to the label.

It is the aim of progressive health-conscious countries to raise the standard of milk production, so that all will be produced from tuberculin-free cows.

Channel Island Milk.—Milk from Jersey and Guernsey cows has an especially high fat content, hence it is rich in cream. The farmer producing such milk is allowed to label it " Channel Island Milk " provided it contains not less than 4 per cent. butter fat. It is slightly more expensive. This milk may also be Tuberculin Tested, Pasteurised or both.

SUMMARY

DISEASES SPREAD BY MILK

(1) *From the cow.*

(a) Bovine tuberculosis.

(b) Streptococcal infections.

(c) Undulant fever.

(2) *From the milker, or anyone handling the milk.*

(a) Enteric infections, e.g. typhoid and paratyphoid fever.

(b) Dysentery.

(c) Diphtheria.

(d) Staphylococcal infections.

(e) Streptococcal infections.

(f) Tuberculosis.

(3) *From contaminated utensils used in process of milking and distribution; most probably contaminated by carelessness, inefficient sterilisation, or by washing with polluted water.*

(a) Streptococcal or Staphylococcal infections.

(b) Enteric infections—typhoid, dysentery, etc.

(c) Parasitic worms.

(4) *In transit and particularly in the home, by exposure to dust, flies, dirty utensils and infected humans and rodents.*

All those diseases already mentioned in Groups (2) and (3).

FOOD POISONING AND INFECTIONS SPREAD BY FOOD

This subject has considerably exercised the Health Authorities for many years, and although at present alimentary infections conveyed by food, water and milk are known to be preventable by various community health measures, epidemics and outbreaks of food poisoning are still a matter of concern. Obviously, there are extremes of seriousness in disease and poisoning; at one end are severe enteric fevers, e.g., typhoid and botulism, and at the other, mild diarrhœa and vomiting. The severe end of the scale has been reduced to an occasional outbreak which gives rise to great publicity and high-level investigation and control—at the mild end thousands of cases of slight food poisoning are not treated by the doctor, and therefore are not diagnosed or notified. In spite of this, and of all our knowledge of the causes of food poisoning, several thousand cases are notified to Community Physicians each year.

This seems a grave admission, but there are many reasons for it. Our feeding habits have changed; the development of school meals services, factory canteens, local authority restaurants, and so on, has resulted in a great increase in communal feeding. This and other things have probably resulted in a change of social habit, with many more people eating away from home. All this requires mass preparation and serving. Many more people handle the food before it is eaten, and much food is pooled. The result of this is obvious. The mistake or carelessness of one person may affect a large number of people, either because he is handling a lot of food or because the small amount he handles is pooled with the rest. Business monopolies and better forms of transport have also widened the distribution of food. On the other hand, this in itself should have improved the standard of preparation.

The term " Bacterial Food Poisoning " or simply " Food Poisoning " usually means acute gastro-enteritis due to the swallowing of food containing certain bacteria *or* their pre-formed toxins, in sufficient amount to make them irritant to the mucosa of the stomach and small intestine. It should be distinguished from bacterial infection.

Bacterial infection—caused by ingestion of contaminated food and leading to diseases such as typhoid—and *bacterial food poisoning*, are not always clearly distinguishable. The same organism may cause one or the other in different conditions (e.g. salmonellae in food usually cause gastro-enteritis, but sometimes they cause an *infection* in which the germ actually invades the tissues and gives rise to a type of " enteric fever ").

Bacterial Food Poisoning—Two Types. (*a*) Infection type— the incubation period for which is 4–36 hours. Probably the bacteria multiply to some extent in the alimentary canal. (*b*) Toxin type—the incubation period for which is shorter—1–6 hours or occasionally as long as 18 hours. The attack is usually sharper with more vomiting and prostration.

(Old " Ptomaine Theory "—Ptomaine are organic nitrogen compounds, found in putrefying food.)

Morbidity—the attack rate varies, but tends to be high.

Mortality—is low (except in Botulism).

Bacteriology.

(1) **Salmonella Group.**—Some hundreds of varieties are known, the majority coming originally from animals and birds (rats, mice, ducks and hens, cows, pigs, etc.).

The common vehicles are all meats, especially " made up " dishes, milk and cream, eggs (from ducks, particularly) and egg products. (It is rare in canned meat, except ham.) *N.B.* The food usually looks normal.

(2) **Staphylococci** (some strains only). **Toxin Type only.** *Source of Staphylococci.*—Septic cuts and sores; noses and skins of carriers. These are hard to exclude, so one must rely on the prevention of multiplication.

(3) **Clostridium Welchii**—from meat and gravy. Spores are present in the meat; these spores may resist cooking and if meat and gravy are kept warm, they multiply in the anærobic conditions created by a " blanket " of fat and meat particles.

(4) **Non-specific Bacteria** (ordinarily non-pathogenic). *Proteus, Bacterium Coli.*—Some strains, if they multiply in food, may give rise to the toxin type of food poisoning.

(5) **Botulism** (*Botulus*, a sausage). This is an intoxication, not an infection—the *Clostridium botulinum* (*B. Botulinus*). The spores are heat-resistant, widely distributed in soil, and are strict anærobes. They dislike acid foods (fruit, etc.). Botulism is caused by inadequately heated canned or bottled foods (which are therefore free from oxygen), and particularly if they are not acid. It is usually due to *home canning*. It is often fatal but now fortunately rare. The food looks sound. An antitoxin has been prepared but is not generally successful.

Mode of Contamination of Food.

(1) By the animal or bird from which the meat or eggs came.

(2) By rats and mice, by human sufferers or carriers of salmonella (e.g., mild ambulant cases).

Factors in Size of Dose. Probably a few salmonellae can be ingested harmlessly. The minimum infecting dose varies from one salmonella to another, from hundreds of thousands to millions. More virulent bacteria, which may cause infection of the alimentary tract, need fewer to cause diseases (e.g. typhoid and cholera). Therefore, fresh food, correct storage, refrigeration, are all important factors.

PREVENTION OF BACTERIAL FOOD POISONING

Main points to remember:

(1) *Healthy Animals.*—The rearing of healthy animals, the maintenance and supervision of hygienic slaughterhouses, and regular meat inspection are all important in preventing food poisoning.

(2) *The Supervision of Food Handlers.*—This applies particularly to those working in communal kitchens and food stores. People who are known typhoid carriers must be excluded from handling food at any stage. Anyone suffering from diarrhœa and/or vomiting— however mild—should be encouraged to report to the doctor, and prevented from handling food. All personnel should be given proper facilities for hand-washing after going to the lavatory, and encouraged to make use of them. All cooks should be taught the importance of the thorough cooking of foodstuffs likely to cause food poisoning, e.g. duck eggs, meat dishes—especially when it is reheated as in rissoles, brawn, etc.

(3) *The Value of Refrigeration.*—Although cold does not destroy organisms, it does render them inactive.

Frozen chicken and other poultry need to be thoroughly thawed and must be sufficiently heated (cooked) to kill the Salmanella that may be in the deepest parts.

(4) *Elimination of flies, rodents, etc.*—Those responsible for food stores or food preparation should know the danger of food contamination by flies, insects and rodents. All such creatures should be vigorously attacked and destroyed, and their breeding grounds eliminated. Food of all kinds should be protected from them.

(5) *Reliable Food.*—Buy meat, fish and other food from reliable sources; do not take risks by eating food that looks or smells doubtful,

although it must be remembered that food causing infections often looks, smells and tastes normal.

It is also wise to remember that pet foods can be dangerous. Separate equipment is advised and these foods segregated from humans food. Hands should be washed thoroughly after handling pet meat.

(6) *Special Care when Catering for Infants and Children.*—It is important to be especially careful when catering for infants and young children, or for any child who is or has been ill. This particularly applies in warm weather, when flies are more active. Gastro-enteritis in infants is still a killing disease. It is also wise to exercise special care when catering for groups of children and adolescents on holiday, at school, at Guide camps, etc. Be certain to use a reliable source of water.

(7) *Care of Kitchen and Cooking Utensils.*—It is important to keep the kitchen and cooking utensils clean and in good condition. If you are a housewife, insist on a good standard of personal hygiene for yourself, your family, and for those responsible for preparing, conveying and serving food. Set your family a good example.

(8) *In the event of suspected food poisoning, notify the doctor;* be as helpful as possible by giving clear and correct information and keeping any food left over, in case it is needed for bacterial examination.

If you are a nurse, remember you are a teacher of healthy living. Set other people a good example and take every opportunity to teach others the importance of clean food.

Moulds and Yeasts. Other factors which spoil food, but do not actually cause infection or poisoning, are moulds or yeasts. These spread by forming spores, but although they spoil a good deal of food they are not really dangerous to health. By their growing they do not produce toxins as other organisms tend to do. The food smells and looks unpleasant so it is not likely to be eaten. Moulds grow particularly well on bread, cheese, fruit and meat, etc., and quickly cause decomposition. Many moulds are used to advantage, especially in cheese making.

Sir Alexander Fleming made one of the greatest discoveries of this century by realising that the growth of a certain type of mould (penicillium) inhibited the activity of micro-organisms.

Yeast cells also spoil certain commodities, without causing poisoning. It is yeast which brings about the fermentation in wine making, etc. Louis Pasteur did some interesting work in this connection, and paved the way for the work of Lister in antiseptic surgery.

HOUSING IN RELATION TO HEALTH

A study of the nineteenth-century history of this country provides evidence to show the strong connection between housing and health. Four serious diseases, such as typhus, cholera, tuberculosis and acute rheumatism, would make a most interesting study of this connection. Medical statisticians have produced some convincing figures to show the relationship.

The industrial revolution of the early nineteenth century, while undoubtedly responsible for the economic survival of this country, was also responsible for the most appalling insanitary and over-crowded housing conditions. The slums which still disgrace our industrial cities originate in that period. Factory workers were crowded into homes cheaply and hastily built on unsatisfactory sites, with unsatisfactory water supplies and defective sanitation. Because coal was the main source of power, the plight of the people living in these densely populated areas was made worse by the constant pall of smoke which vitiated the atmosphere.

The success and development of our industries made matters worse; people moved in from the rural areas, attracted from the land to the factory by higher wages, into housing areas already over-crowded. Factories were designed primarily to produce goods, with little thought given to conditions and their effect on health. There were no laws governing the employment of child labour; conditions in the mines were unbelievably primitive; and wages, although better than in agriculture, were incredibly small. Intoxicating liquor was cheap, moral and ethical standards were low, and educa-tion and birth control were non-existent.

Louis Pasteur and Joseph Lister had only just begun their work. There was little or no understanding of the cause of disease, or of its prevention. Vitamins were unknown and supplies of fresh fruit and vegetables were available only to the wealthy. All these factors created a vicious circle which resulted in poverty and ill-health of every kind; one cannot single out any special factor as being more responsible than others, but undoubtedly poor housing was one of the most important.

Since the London Building Act of 1894, many Acts of Parliament have been passed, notably the Housing Acts of 1919, 1936 and 1957, and more recently the Town and Country Planning Acts 1944–1959, and the New Towns Act 1946. The development of housing management schemes pioneered by Octavia Hill, and the attention now being directed to this problem by the Local Authori-ties, has done much to improve the situation, but we are all very conscious of the amount there is still to do. Two world wars have imposed serious setbacks, not only by causing the destruction of many habitable dwellings, but by preventing the progress of slum clearance schemes and the repair of existing houses. In spite of life lost during the Second World War, the population has steadily increased and, much more importantly, the number of families has increased and the average age of marriage has decreased. There has also been a steady flow of refugees and immigrants from all over the world.

During most of the nineteenth century, the heavy death toll and low expectation of life was the result of a great number of diseases. Those affecting the alimentary tract, e.g. cholera, typhoid and paratyphoid fever, dysentery, summer diarrhœa and vomiting, and intestinal worms could be mainly attributed to lack of or poor sanitation and unsafe water supplies. Diseases affecting the respiratory system were spread by direct contact and droplet infection and, therefore, aggravated by overcrowding, e.g. tuberculosis, diphtheria and streptococcal infections of all kinds. Deficiency diseases, e.g. rickets and scurvy, were caused by lack of sunshine, and lack of vitamins in a poor diet. Typhus and smallpox were still prevalent, and all those numerous diseases which result from overcrowding. Lowered resistance and lack of vitality favoured the spread of tetanus, gas-gangrene, erysipelas, puerperal sepsis, etc. In addition one must not forget that the spread of venereal disease is encouraged by low moral standards and aggravated by overcrowding. These conditions not only took a heavy toll of life, but caused a high level of morbidity. The later results of rickets, combined with the high incidence of sepsis and the general low state of nutrition and vitality, were amongst the many causes of a high maternal and infant mortality rate.

Many of these diseases, notably smallpox and diphtheria, have been overcome by vaccination and immunisation; other serious ones e.g. cholera and the more serious enteric diseases, by improved water and sanitary conditions. Better nutrition, knowledge and use of vitamins and knowledge of the value of fresh air and sunshine have almost eradicated deficiency diseases—e.g., rickets is now a rarity. In our generation and the next, little should be seen of their after effects.

Those diseases still occurring and causing considerable mortality rates are not thought to be largely attributable to poor housing. One must, therefore, remember that other factors must be considered also; faulty nutrition and a low standard of personal care generally.

Diseases such as acute rheumatism and tuberculosis still occur in children of the higher social grades, despite every care.

Both these diseases carry a high morbidity rate, and are especially aggravated by overcrowded and damp living conditions. The combined efforts of the Public Health and Housing Authorities have done much to bring about a definite statistical improvement. Medical science must also share the credit. Improved methods of diagnosis, combined with the therapeutic results of the sulphonamide and antibiotic groups of drugs, and the prophylactic use of B.C.G. have combined to bring about this improvement. Many tuberculosis beds are now empty, and the incidence of cardiac invalidism which resulted from acute rheumatism is steadily declining owing to the control of streptococcal infection. The compulsory notification of disease and the pasteurisation of milk must necessarily share the credit.

All this sounds very satisfactory. What then is the present state of affairs with regard to housing? One of the few good things that came out of the last war was that it probably forced the hands of many Borough and District Councils to make radical slum clearance a reality. Bombing destroyed many overcrowded industrial areas and made many others uninhabitable. This has resulted in tremendous redevelopment schemes to house the working population in estates comprised of houses, flats, shops and community centres. In fact, whole communities on the borders of the cities have been built up where families can enjoy the fresh air and open spaces of the countryside. The Government has laid down definite specifications: back-to-back houses are prohibited, roads must be of a certain width, yard space and garden space around houses must not be less than a certain area. In the cities, large new blocks of flats are being erected to house people who prefer to stay there, but, as with the housing estates, there must be adequate space provided for children to play and fresh air to circulate.

How has all this change affected health? Each generation seems to develop its own problems, and diseases developing from our modern way of life tend to be different from those of our ancestors. Psychosomatic disease and mental breakdowns caused by stress and strain are taking the place of the infections and physical illnesses of former years with one or two exceptions, e.g. poliomyelitis. The breadwinner is always striving, sometimes beyond his capacity, to provide the means of living in an attractive house, fitted with all available modern conveniences. Stress may result when both husband and wife work full time, and this sometimes tends to cause domestic tension. Material comforts and modern equipment is so easy to obtain on the instalment system that some families cannot resist the temptation to get themselves involved in financial commitments far beyond their means. All may be well while the couple are able to work, but the arrival of children, illness or unemployment are the beginning of family tension which may well result in mental or physical breakdown.

Other problems affecting health are those which result from the break-up of families. Members are moved away into housing estates and family cohesion is broken by distance. There is a tendency for members of the family to lose contact with each other. There is an odd inclination in families moved from tenements to housing estates to want to " keep themselves to themselves "; troubles are not shared and there is not the same tendency for neighbours or relatives to offer help during confinement and illness. Loneliness is becoming a very real thing, affecting not only the elderly but also the young. Loneliness on a housing estate can be much worse than that suffered in some remote village in the country. All this adds to the strain of living, and in many cases mental and physical breakdown can be indirectly attributed to it.

Houses inconveniently planned may also contribute to strain, e.g. those with lack of storage space or inadequate drying facilities and cooking arrangements.

Before leaving this subject of housing in relation to health, one should not overlook the physical danger to which the individual is subjected in a modern house. There was something to be said for the four simple walls and roof which primitive men lived in; they gained shelter from the external elements but had no modern luxuries to enjoy. On the other hand, there were fewer dangers. Many people will be surprised to know that a recent four-year survey showed that in this country for every four fatal accidents on the roads five occurred in the home. The hazards of the modern house are many, particularly to those very young and old, and to those of subnormal intelligence. Unguarded fires of all sorts, particularly gas and electric; worn, faulty or amateur electric wiring, exposed gas taps accessible to little children, are extremely dangerous. Frayed mats, trailing flexes, highly polished floors, ill-lighted passages and stairs are a menace to elderly folk. Teapots, kettles, saucepans, trailing tablecloths, etc., are a constant source of danger to little children. Badly placed medicine cupboards, bottles of disinfectant or weed-killer left about, are from time to time responsible for deaths of children or for their disablement. Modern domestic gadgets are also a physical danger—electric washing machines and presses, vacuum cleaners, washing-up machines, electric irons, pressure cookers, etc., all need to be understood.

While the many plastic gadgets are a great boon, they also present new dangers. Plastic sheeting and bags left around are highly dangerous to children and animals, and recently attention has been

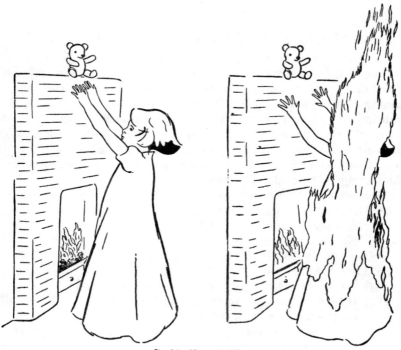

Fig. 24.   Unguarded Fire.

focused on the modern carry-cot. The average design at present, with unventilated base and surrounds, exposes an infant or small baby to risk of suffocation. This may occur if the baby gets in a position with face downwards, and particularly if he vomits or regurgitates food. The mattress, being in the well of the cot, also causes decreased oxygen content of the surrounding air and this aggravates the situation. Recently, coroners have urged that carry-cot design should receive urgent attention.

In spite of these disadvantages improved housing schemes can claim a good deal of the credit for the improvement in life statistics shown between the years 1900–1947. The crude death rate has fallen by 31 per cent. The expectation of life has increased by 16 years for females and 18 years for males. The infant death rate has fallen from 150 to under 30 per 1,000 live births. Typhus has disappeared, smallpox, typhoid fever and diphtheria have almost disappeared. Most infectious diseases can now be prevented or controlled; notifications for tuberculosis and rheumatism are rapidly declining, and poliomyelitis has almost disappeared.

MINIMUM REQUIREMENTS FOR HEALTH

In a temperate climate such as ours, a dwelling house must be somewhat elaborate. It must be built to protect the inhabitants from the elements and to be really comfortable it must render them almost independent of them. It must in no way be responsible for causing disease by poor structure, condition, or lack of facilities: and in its simplest sense this is possibly all a dwelling house need do. But this is not sufficient for modern needs, which demand accommodation to *promote health*, i.e. give a positive state of well-being that is something far beyond mere absence of disease.

The recommended Standards of Fitness for Habitation which were laid down in 1946 were as follows.

The dwelling should:

(1) Be in all respects dry.
(2) Be in a good state of repair.
(3) Have each room properly lighted and ventilated.
(4) Have an adequate supply of wholesome water laid on for all purposes inside the dwelling.
(5) Be provided with efficient and adequate means of supplying hot water for domestic purposes.
(6) Have an internal or otherwise readily accessible water closet.
(7) Have a fixed bath, preferably in a separate room.
(8) Have a proper drainage system.
(9) Be provided with adequate points for artificial lighting in each room.
(10) Be provided with adequate facilities for heating each habitable room.
(11) Have satisfactory facilities for preparing and cooking food.
(12) Have a well-ventilated larder or food store.
(13) Have a proper provision for the storage of fuel.
(14) Have a satisfactory surfaced path to outbuildings and convenient access from a street to the back door.

This was considered a reasonable standard to be aimed at when building new houses, and in this country should present no real difficulty. There is considerable difficulty, however, in trying to bring the standards of old houses up to modern requirements. Sometimes it is quite impossible, particularly in country districts; and housing programmes are so controlled by the supply of raw materials, labour and money, that many old houses must go on being inhabited.

It is difficult to state anything more definite about minimum requirements for health, for so much depends on the " housekeeper ". An educated, sensible, intelligent person can keep herself and her family healthy in a house with the most limited facilities. Conversely, a modern house can quickly become an insanitary and unhealthy dwelling if badly managed. It is said by some, indeed, that new housing estates will not bring about any improvement in the standards of living of families from slum areas. This is not necessarily so. It has been proved without doubt that the majority of families, if given reasonable living accommodation, will strive to improve their standards to the level of their accommodation. Problem families still exist, probably always will, but in the minority.

Point 10 of the recommended standards needs special attention. It is all very well to suggest " each room should be provided with adequate facilities for heating ". As a civilised country we are far behind in this respect—the facilities provided to heat the rooms of houses now being built are usually electric points to take a fire, or an electric fire built into the wall. These are not only often dangerous to children and old people, but far too expensive for the average working-class family. We have not yet faced up to the challenge to provide proper space heating in our houses, so that all rooms can be fully used, both in summer and winter. It is very difficult for children, particularly if they are trying to keep up a Grammar School standard, to have to study and do homework in the living room, which in many cases is also the kitchen. And often this is so because it is the only warm room, or even the only living room. Television has made this problem worse—the whole family tends to concentrate in the one room that is warm and contains the television set. As a community living in such a climate as ours, we should strive for better insulation of houses, compulsory facilities for space heating, and better plumbing arrangements, so that a hard winter is not so expensive and disastrous for the householder. We know all these facts, but how slow we are putting them into operation.

A well-designed, well-equipped house may become unfit for habitation if it is allowed to become:

(1) Overcrowded.

(2) In a state of disrepair—so that it becomes damp or unsafe.

(3) Infested with rodents, vermin and parasites.

(4) Insanitary.

Because of our climate dampness is a big problem in this country. A house may become damp because it is built on an unsatisfactory site, or has an inadequate or defective damp proof course. Dampness may also be caused by defective external brickwork or roof.

Houses allowed to fall into a state of disrepair not only become damp, but are likely to become infested with rodents and vermin. The occupants, who usually have poor standards of personal hygiene, also become infested with parasites. The whole state of affairs quickly deteriorates and the dreary picture of a problem family will be the result.

Local Authorities in the U.K. are encouraged to make grants to enable old houses to be improved and brought up to modern standards. They are also allowed to offer Council houses for sale. At present the Local Authorities own over four million houses and flats. This represents a quarter of the United Kingdom's housing stock.

The Local Authority has the right to declare a house unfit for human habitation if:

(1) It is in such a state of disrepair that it cannot be put right at reasonable cost.

(2) It is overcrowded.

(3) It is insanitary.

For more technical information on house construction the reader should refer to a more detailed textbook.

OVERCROWDING

The Housing Act of 1936 was the first Act which really attempted to define overcrowding. It is a problem that concerns not only the Local Authority of a city—it is just as likely to occur in the small country cottage.

Laws regarding overcrowding aim at providing adequate separate sleeping accommodation for the sexes, and lays down definite standards relating to occupants in ratio to numbers of rooms and floor areas. The word " room " applies to living and sleeping rooms, but does not include bathroom, scullery, kitchen or any room with a floor space of less than 50 sq. ft. A child under one year old is not taken into account, and a child between the age of one and ten years is counted as half a unit.

For further details the reader must refer to a more comprehensive textbook. For a general understanding it is sufficient to know that a two-roomed house is considered suitable for three persons, and a three-roomed house for five. If a house is found by the Health Authority to be overcrowded the landlord is held responsible and warning is given to the tenant. If this warning is disregarded an eviction order may be served and the tenancy terminated.

Overcrowding is closely related to the spread of infectious disease, including tuberculosis. It is responsible for lowering moral standards, particularly with regard to children and adolescents. Mental breakdown can also be attributed to it.

Movable Dwellings. A number of people, for reasons of personal choice or necessity, live permanently or temporarily in dwellings other than permanent houses. This term is used to include caravans, tents or huts, used both by day and night for human occupation. The law provides for them and makes provision not only for the welfare and personal health of the dwellers, but also for the safety of the community. The inhabitants of a movable dwelling must have access to a safe water supply, and must have suitable sanitary provision for the disposal of refuse. The dwelling must be kept reasonably clean and properly ventilated and must not be overcrowded. There are usually special by-laws relating to the accommodation provided for families, e.g. hop pickers, who live in such dwellings for seasonal work. Provision is also made for the education of children of school age.

A few people live in canal boats, but only if the vessel is properly registered and considered by law to provide suitable and sanitary accommodation. There must be proper sleeping accommodation, adequate ventilation and sufficient supply of wholesome water. These dwellings must be open for inspection by duly authorised officers.

Common Lodging Houses. There are people who, for reasons of choice or circumstances, have no fixed abodes, and depend for shelter on what is called a common lodging house. The law controls these dwellings also, and each one must be registered with the Local Authority. A section of the Public Health Act 1936 and by-laws require adequate spacing to be allowed for sleeping, the sexes to be segregated, and feeding and washing facilities to be adequate to prevent the incidence or spread of disease. Water supply and sanitary arrangements must also be satisfactory and bedding and bedclothes properly cleaned.

CARE OF THE HOME

Of all the definitions for " home ", the one most appropriate is: " A charitable abode ", " A place where one is at ease and familiar " and no book on personal and communal health can be complete without containing something on one of the most important factors in the promotion of positive health.

So far in this section on housing only the material aspect has been considered, but of what value is a beautifully kept house, with more than minimum requirements for health, if it does not fulfil the purpose of being a real home? This is of the utmost importance to children and quite important to people of all ages, although adults safely grown to maturity would probably suffer less. It is, however, true that no one, however stable, will really enjoy positive health and perform good work if the home side of life is at fault.

More than ever before the older generation must do everything possible to impress this on the younger generation. The basis of home is built on the relationship that exists between the parents. However humble the home may be, it is the little things that matter to children. The family that can share its sorrows, problems and pleasures, and express them in tears of sorrow or hugs of real affection and pleasure, has got something very real. The real home means so much to children; everyone round the same table, enjoying a meal that mother or father has cooked, the evening bath, bedtime story, prayers and a goodnight kiss. A special cupboard or box, or some corner where a child can keep his toys and treasures, and so often the most simple and inexpensive toys are those which give the most pleasure; an orange box with a curtain round makes an admirable locker for a small boy or girl. In the right sort of home it is a long while before the growing child ceases to experience pleasure in coming home to renew acquaintance with old special toys and possibly a cat or dog.

To fulfil its function properly the home must be the one place where a child can really express his feelings, so aiding his emotional development. The best parents are those prepared to be fought, defied, loved and hated, but they are the people who can stand it. A child from this type of home usually enjoys school and looks upon it as a place of organisation and discipline, whereas a child who is too disciplined or unhappy at home will be more likely to give trouble at school.

Once having established a real home, its care should be the responsibility of the whole family. The building itself should be kept in good repair; the quick correction of minor faults will often prevent the need for major repairs. Gutters should be kept free of debris— they often require cleaning after leaves fall in the autumn. Children can be taught to appreciate, enjoy and care for a garden; and a supply of flowers for the home is a great advantage. Inside the home, furniture, however simple and primitive, should be cared for and kept clean. Windows should be kept clean and clear of furniture, etc. Chimneys need regular sweeping. Rubbish, grubby clothes, food, etc., should not be allowed to accumulate, and cupboards and carpets need periodic moving to keep them free from dust. Fresh air should be allowed to circulate.

Nowadays, house decorations are a major expense, but again much can be done to brighten a house. We have such a wonderful variety of colours and materials to choose from. The outside of the house needs repainting about every 3–5 years, and the inside according to the amount it is used, and by whom it is used.

For more detailed knowledge of house care, the reader must refer to a good housekeeping book. Above all, it is important to remember that it is the atmosphere of welcome and friendliness as well as cleanliness which makes a happy successful home. A place where children and parents feel safe, can find affection, comfort and good counsel; a place where the visitor and the stranger will find a real welcome—the offer of a cup of tea after a journey, or to the casual caller, is often a good indication of the generosity of the householder.

HOUSEHOLD PESTS AND VERMIN

Many of these have been dealt with in the section on Personal Health. There are a few, however, not yet mentioned. Most can be prevented or eradicated by relatively simple measures. The pest control section of the Local Authority will assist the householder if it is necessary. Whatever method is adopted it must be intelligently and carefully carried out—the best insecticides will fail if slipshod methods are used.

Insects.

(1) *Fleas and Bed Bugs.*—See Personal Health.

(2) *Ants.*—There are two types of ant. House ants are those which breed in houses and will sometimes prove a nuisance in the kitchen and larder. Garden ants normally live out of doors, but will occasionally enter houses. With both types, efforts should be made to find the nest and destroy it. House ants can be destroyed by using a special bait or spray, which must be carefully used with the assistance of the Local Authority. Garden ants can be discouraged from entering the house by painting a band of tanglefoot around the house below all openings where the ants could enter. It need not be more than one inch wide, but must be kept " tacky". Gammaxene powder sprinkled round the house may also be effective. Nests are destroyed with boiling water or insecticides.

Cockroaches.—These tend to collect in old buildings centrally heated, and around the brickwork of old ovens. They are difficult to get rid of. DDT* powder or Gammaxene can be blown into all cracks and crevices. DDT emulsion can be painted in bands on a non-absorbent surface, and a special spray can be used to force the emulsion into cracks and crevices. All food should be carefully protected and breeding grounds energetically attacked.

Silver Fish and Crickets.—Both these insects are relatively harmless and are, in fact, good scavengers. Occasionally the latter may prove a nuisance by creating a noise and can be destroyed by insecticides.

Wasps are a nuisance during the fruit season; jam and all sweet things should be kept covered and nests destroyed. Particular care should be taken with children. A sting on the tongue or throat can be dangerous.

Clothes Moths.—These do not endanger health, but can prove an expensive nuisance. Particular care should be taken at the end of the winter season when putting away extra blankets and woollen clothes. It is best to have them cleaned or washed. If they should be stained with food or body secretions, particularly sweat, they will form an ideal breeding ground for the clothes moth. An effort should be made to keep trunks, boxes and cupboards, etc., as moth-proof as possible. Various moth-proof containers are available, and many types of moth brick. In addition to all these, cleanliness and fresh air are good deterrents. Manufacturers are now developing methods for moth-proofing woollen materials, and some firms claim to do this when cleaning articles. When buying carpets and placing heavy

* DDT, while effective, is discouraged because of its persistent nature and subsequent danger.

furniture, it is wise to sprinkle DDT along the felt under the edges of the carpet and under any heavy furniture that cannot be easily moved for cleaning.

Flies in this country are a constant menace to health. They are not only a personal nuisance but they infect food and by so doing spread disease. There are many beside the common house fly—the green and blue bottle, the stable fly—all are dangerous to mankind because of their dirty habits. Flies breed at an alarming rate on any dung heap or dirt. For this reason they should be kept out of the house and away from food. It is said that the offspring from one fly may number 432,000 in seven weeks. Between May and September particularly flies spread disease wherever they go. They particularly like sugar, meat, fish, cheese, butter, milk and bread. Germs are carried on their sticky feet, and to make matters worse, excreta, saliva and vomit is deposited on the food to dissolve it. Flies spread dysentery, summer diarrhœa-and-vomiting, and probably poliomyelitis.

All flies should be destroyed by DDT sprays, flypaper and swats. Breeding grounds should be eliminated, all food kept covered. The larder window should be protected by a fine wire gauze screen, and the larder door kept tightly closed. The house should be kept clean.

If babies are in the house, soiled napkins, whether wet or dirty, should not be left exposed, but put immediately into a bucket with a well-fitting lid.

Spiders, daddy-long-legs and other insects inhabit most houses but are much more likely to be a nuisance in those with thatched roofs. Although they do no harm it is best to discourage them. Spiders will spin their webs in any corner, behind any picture or cupboard and around the light flexes. The web is made to trap flies and other insects. Regular high dusting and spring cleaning, i.e. periodic cleaning behind boxes and cupboards, is necessary to eliminate these insects.

For this reason the built-in type of cupboard for books, clothes, etc., is becoming more popular. The traditional type of wardrobe is difficult to move and always proves a dust trap on the top.

Rodents. *Rats* are rodents that cause a lot of trouble, particularly in ports and warehouses. They will infest premises if food is left accessible to them. By their gnawing they may imperil the foundations of buildings, damage water pipes, electric cables and other fittings. They attack textiles and consume and foul food. Although rats in this country are not common in dwelling houses, they inhabit warehouses in vast numbers, and every effort should be made to destroy them. There are two main types of rats—brown and black. The brown is the sewer type, which feeds on filth and lives in the drainage systems. Rats breed from March to August, and it is possible for one pair to give rise to more than 1,000 offspring during one single breeding season.

Rats can carry specific diseases, although this is now uncommon in this country. They are often responsible, however, for spreading bacterial food poisoning. Every effort should be made to repair buildings and stop up holes. Accumulation of refuse should be avoided, all rubbish and waste food bins should have well-fitting lids. If the problem is serious it may be necessary to have the expert assistance of the local Rodent Officer, or a few rats may be destroyed by trapping or poisoning. Traps are best set lightly at right angles to the run, the runways being determined by droppings. In both cases, great care must be exercised to ensure the safety of children and domestic pets—most rat poisons are lethal. A disadvantage of poisoning is that the animal, whether rat or mouse, may die in a place which is inaccessible.

Mice.—These are much more common in dwelling houses, particularly in those old or in the country. Mice also can destroy woodwork and fabrics, and damage or infect food. Holes should be stopped up, woodwork repaired and all food kept in safe store cupboards. Mice are destroyed in the same way as rats. A cat, provided it is a good mouser, is an asset.

Insects which affect Timber. *Death Watch Beetle.*—This insect may attack old timber, particularly if it is damp and poorly ventilated. Therefore it is more often found in old houses. The beetles can be recognised by their leaving large bun-shaped pellets in the bore dust produced by the grub, or by exposing themselves on the floor during the period between April and June. Vigorous treatment should be carried out between March and September, but it is very difficult. Infested wood should be removed and bore dust and debris vacuumed. Expert advice should be obtained as this condition is likely to spread.

Lyctus or Powder Beetles.—These insects are able to fly, therefore their range of attack is considerable. The grubs tunnel in sap wood, reducing it to a fine dust. This infestation is best avoided by the elimination of sap wood from all timber used for building and furniture. Where infestation has occurred, infested wood should be removed if possible. If not, treatment with the proper insecticide may be effective. Expert advice should be obtained.

Common Furniture Beetle.—This insect is also able to fly, and normally lives out of doors in dead or dying parts of trees. It does, however, prove a distinct nuisance to the householder when it attacks furniture and structural timbers. The dust produced by the grub contains oval or cylindrical pellets. Energetic and careful treatment is required to destroy these insects, and several applications are necessary. The dust should be removed by a vacuum cleaner and unpolished furniture may be treated with paraffin or turpentine. Where colour is of no importance hot creosote is good. For polished furniture a proprietary insecticide should be used. Applications are preferably made during late spring and early summer, care being taken to deal with all cracks, joints, backs and undersides. Treatment should be repeated several times and for at least two years.

Careful inspection of second-hand furniture should be made before introducing it among other furniture. Active infestation can be ascertained by finding fresh wood dust in the grub holes.

Dry Rot in Wood. This is the decay of wood caused by a fungus. The method of curing this will depend on the type, but expert advice should be obtained. It is likely to occur in the woodwork of old houses, particularly if they are damp or have been standing empty. Treatment is drastic. All affected timber must be removed and burned, timber used for replacement must be treated with a preservative, and the cause of dampness eradicated. If the disease is very extensive the whole property may have to be destroyed, either because it has become unsafe or the cost of treating and repairing the property is out of proportion to its value. This condition may be largely prevented by the insertion of an effective damp-proof course, the use of properly seasoned wood, or the use of wood which is naturally resistant.

For the avoidance of dry rot in timber floors, the most important structural point is to prevent ground moisture rising into the building—this is probably the chief cause of dry rot in floors. The ground is in effect an inexhaustible reservoir from which moisture can rise. This does not apply to floors insulated by air beneath, except in so far as they rest on brick foundations.

Rising damp can be prevented by the inclusion of a damp-proof course at an appropriate position in the building. If this course, which should be impervious to moisture both in the liquid and the vapour form, extends without a break over the whole of the site of the building, no dampness due to ground moisture is possible.

Before property is bought, particularly if it is old, the professional advice of an Architect Surveyor should be obtained.

Creeping Plants—Magnolia, Clematis, Virginia Creeper, etc.—While these may be very attractive, and probably relatively harmless while young, they can cause damage to the structure of a house if allowed to become too well established. The suckers tend to grow into the joints and extract moisture from the cement, reducing it to a powder. Insects may become more common in the house, and rats and mice may enter. Birds nesting may also prove a nuisance as well as damage the fabric of the house. The roots of the plants also may do severe damage by undermining the foundations of the building and even displacing the floor. It must be remembered that the amount of growth under a bush is equivalent to that above ground. While the latter may be clipped back, the roots will continue to grow unless properly controlled. Wall creepers may be the cause of dampness.

Birds Nesting.—Starlings which nest under the eaves should be discouraged. They tend to find their way into the attics of the house and often damage the fabric with nesting activity, and are rather unhygienic. Jackdaws also cause considerable damage. If there is any evidence of their attempting to build in the chimneys a protecting wire mesh screen should be used. Once jackdaws have become established, sticks, straw and debris will be taken down the chimney for the nest. They will cause obvious trouble and cannot be removed easily. Efforts with the usual brush or vacuum sweeper are usually ineffective, and they are often difficult to remove from above. The law prohibits smoking the nest out or setting fire to it for obvious reasons of nuisance and risk of fire, so it may mean having to dismantle the chimney.

Dirt.—It was Louis Pasteur who proved that there was no spontaneous generation of life, so we do not believe that " dirt can grow legs ", but we do know that dirt and disease go together. Dirt can be said to be the best friend of disease and the constant enemy of man. Bugs, lice, fleas and bacteria flourish in dirty surroundings. They do not survive long in clean ones. Soap and water and fresh air are the best deterrents. Spitting in the home or in any public place is dirty, unpleasant and sometimes dangerous. If sputum contains germs these may survive drying and form infected dust. Tuberculosis can be spread in this way. In this country spitting in any public place is prohibited by law.

Litter makes dirty unattractive surroundings, whether in the house, garden or countryside. Empty unwashed food tins, fruit peels, paper, etc., all attract flies and rodents, as well as create an untidy unpleasant appearance.

From an early age, children can be taught to be reasonably clean and tidy, can learn to appreciate cleanliness in their homes, schools and surroundings. The best and most effective way to teach children is to set them a good example.

VENTILATION, HEATING AND LIGHTING

AIR

The *air* is a mixture of gases which surrounds the earth and upon which life is entirely dependent. The most vital constituent of this mixture is oxygen, of which there is approximately 21 per cent. Oxygen is necessary for respiration and combustion. The tissue cells demand a constant supply which reaches them via the air passages, alveoli, and the hæmoglobin in the red blood corpuscles. Nitrogen forms the greater proportion of air, it is not used by the body but serves to dilute the oxygen and other constituents.

The composition of air by volume is approximately:

Nitrogen	79 per cent. (almost)
Oxygen	21 per cent. (almost)
Carbon dioxide	0·03 per cent.
Argon and other rare gases	A trace.
Water vapour	Variable.

Impurities such as suspended particles of soot and dust are present in the air of all towns and cities.

Bacteria to some extent are present everywhere, particularly in the more populated areas.

Ozone is present in the air by the sea.

The temperature varies according to the time of year and nearness to the Equator. The sun's rays pass through the atmosphere and are absorbed by earth and water. The nearer the equator the more intense the heat because the sun's rays strike more densely. The air passes over the earth and water and is warmed by contact. This causes a movement of air because, as it is warmed, the molecules get forced farther apart by their increasing speed, the air becomes lighter and rises and cool air takes its place. As the air rises it again becomes cooler, to fall elsewhere.

TEMPERATURE

The temperature of the air is measured by a thermometer consisting of a fine graduated glass tube containing mercury or alcohol. This liquid expands when heated and contracts when cooled and the graduations may be marked according to the Centigrade (boiling point 100°) or Fahrenheit Scale (boiling point 212°). In this country the temperature on a warm day in the shade is usually between 60°–70°F or 15°–22°C whereas in the winter it may be below freezing point. 65°F or 18°C is considered a comfortable temperature for the air in a living room.

PRESSURE

Pressure is the term used to describe the weight or force that the air exerts on the land at sea-level. It is approximately 15 lb. per square inch. As one climbs above sea-level so the pressure is lessened, conversely as one descends below sea-level so the pressure increases. Atmospheric pressure is measured by a barometer, the most simple of which was made as long ago as 1643 by an Italian, Torricelli. It consisted of a thick-walled glass tube about 33 inches long, sealed at one end and filled with mercury. With all air expelled and the open end of the tube covered with the thumb, it was inverted in a basin of mercury. It was seen that some of the mercury ran out, and after a short while a column of mercury about 30 inches or 76 centimetres high was supported. Mercury is still used for barometers because of its great weight (a lighter substance would need a longer column), and the fact that it runs cleanly up and down the tube, is opaque and easily seen. Moist air is lighter and, therefore, exerts less pressure on the mercury, so that one speaks of the *barometer falling* when wet weather is expected. On the other hand, dry air is heavier, exerts more pressure on the mercury, so supporting a higher column, and the term the mercury is rising indicates that dry weather is expected.

There is a second type of barometer called the *Aneroid barometer*. The word " aneroid " means not moist—in other words it is a type of barometer in which no liquid is used. It consists of a thin metal box, almost exhausted of air. The lid of the box moves in and out as the atmospheric pressure on the outside varies. The movements are indicated by a pointer moving over a dial.

HUMIDITY

Humidity is the term used to describe the amount of water vapour in the air. Water in the form of invisible vapour is always present to some extent. It is evident in clouds, mist, fog and falling rain. It is also seen as condensation on the inside of windows in hot rooms, and on the outside of a glass containing cold liquid which is placed in a hot room.

The amount of water vapour the air can hold depends on the temperature, and at a given temperature the atmosphere can only take up a certain definite amount of water vapour. When this limit is reached the air is said to be saturated. This is called *absolute humidity* and is measured by the amount of water vapour the air contains in grams per cubic foot. Air exhaled from the lungs is saturated, and if breathed on to a cool surface, e.g. a window, a fine film of moisture is seen. Equally, on a very cold day air breathed out from the lungs appears as a fine mist.

The term *relative humidity* is used to describe the amount of water vapour actually in the air at a given temperature compared with the amount it would hold at the same temperature if saturated (saturation being taken as 100). This particular science is described as hygrometry, and the instrument for recording relative humidity is a *hygrometer*. The most simple consists of two thermometers mounted side by side, one with an ordinary dry bulb to record the air temperature, and the other with a bulb surrounded by muslin or cotton draped in cold water, to keep it wet. The temperature registered by the wet bulb is always lower than that of the dry bulb owing to the cooling effect of the evaporation from the wet cloth surrounding it. These two readings used with a special chart will give the relative humidity.

The body is sensitive to humidity, since approximately 30 fluid ounces (560 mls) of water are breathed into the air from the lungs and evaporated from the skin of a healthy person each day. If the atmosphere is dry, evaporation will take place readily. Moist air will tend to prevent the cooling of the body by evaporation, and we have all experienced the uncomfortable feeling of dampness on a warm humid day. The same unpleasant feeling may be experienced in a badly ventilated room when temperature and humidity are high and the air is still.

It is considered that an undue **rise in humidity** is probably one of the most important, if not the greatest cause of discomfort in a badly ventilated room, but it is also uncomfortable if the atmosphere is **too dry.** It is probable that the air in a room should hold about three-quarters of the amount of moisture it is capable of holding.

Because the humidity of the atmosphere affects the rate of evaporation of moisture from the body, it is usual to talk about the cooling power of the air. An instrument, the *katathermometer*, aptly described as a comfort meter, was invented by Sir Leonard Hill, to measure this cooling power and estimate the efficiency of ventilation. There are definite standards of humidity laid down for those doing sedentary work and for those doing heavy physical work.

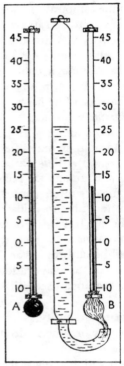

Fig. 25. Hygrometer.
A. Dry bulb.   B. Wet bulb (see text)

IMPURITIES POLLUTING THE ATMOSPHERE

(1) **Respiration.** The air in inhabited places is constantly being polluted by the respiration of humans and animals. As a result of ordinary quiet breathing in an adult about 500 cubic centimetres of air are taken into the lungs and then expelled. The greatest change in this air is that is contains 4 per cent. less oxygen and 4 per cent. more carbon dioxide after being used than before. In addition to this change, the exhaled air is saturated with moisture, is at the temperature of the body, i.e. 37°C (98.4°F) and may contain microorganisms.

It is interesting that in spite of this constant change of oxygen for carbon dioxide, the composition of the atmosphere remains practically constant. This is due to the fact that plants, by day absorb carbon dioxide and liberate oxygen. It is also important to realise that in an ill-ventilated, over-crowded room, although the percentage of oxygen is bound to be decreased below normal and the percentage of carbon dioxide increased by an equivalent amount, *it is not this change which is the main cause of discomfort and ill-effects*. These are due to **increased temperature, excess of moisture** and **lack of air movement,** particularly the latter. Immediate relief is felt if an electric fan is introduced into the room. Because the amount of carbon dioxide in the air is often measured and quoted to indicate the state of the air, it is often wrongly thought to be the main cause of discomfort. This is not so, it is quoted because carbon dioxide is relatively simple to measure, and the amount present is a good indication of the efficiency of the ventilation.

(2) **Combustion Products.** Particularly in towns and cities, impurities resulting from combustion vitiate the atmosphere. The most important factor responsible is the incomplete combustion of coal. In those countries where the enormous resources of energy provided by mountains and water can be converted into electrical power, it is noticeable how fresh and clean is the air. This cleanliness is reflected in the state of the buildings.

Smoke carries poisonous sulphur compounds, tars and carbon monoxide; the sulphur compounds turn into sulphuric acid which attacks buildings, plants and lungs indiscriminately. Smoke in the atmosphere prevents the sun's rays from penetrating, and as much as three-quarters of the sun's energy may be lost as compared with a normal one-half.

Grit, soot and dust are also produced by domestic and industrial fires, and together with the products mentioned above may completely obliterate the sun's rays. As a result in certain conditions a fall in temperature occurs and the atmosphere remains cold. Because it is cold it is still and damp, and the fog becomes gradually more and more unpleasant. The " great smog " of December 1952 was a good example of this process when about 4,000 deaths in the Greater London area were attributed directly to it. In 1956 there was a similar occurrence, although fortunately not so severe. These " smog " conditions were particularly lethal to the very young, the infirm and the elderly.

Various committees were set up to investigate the cause of " smog ", and methods of preventing it, and as a result " The Clean Air Act of 1956 " came into force. As from 20 December 1956 the Local Authority has a statutory duty to enforce certain provisions of this Act, and to make by-laws to prevent air pollution in their particular area. In central London winter sunshine has increased by 70 per cent since 1962.

In brief, the main factors in the prevention of smoke pollution are:

(1) The use of smokeless fuel.

(2) The installation of modern domestic and industrial heating apparatus in all new buildings.

(3) The establishment of smokeless zones or smoke control areas, as in Manchester 1952, London 1955 and elsewhere.

(4) The replacement of obsolete and inefficient heating plants in existing buildings.

(5) Education and training of boiler house staff.

(6) The use of mechanical stokers.

(7) The more widespread use of gas and electricity.

(8) Electrification of railways.

(9) Extraction of grit from industrial furnaces.

(10) The possible use of atomic energy to produce clean heat and power.

(11) The deterrent provided by the power invested in the Local Authority to punish by law persons responsible for creating smoke nuisance.

(12) The provision of Exchequer contributions.

(13) The power of the Local Authority to make grants towards adaptation of fireplaces in all buildings used by charities, etc.

The last two points have particular relevance to the Clean Air Acts of 1956 and 1968. By the end of 1973 about 6.3 million dwellings and commercial premises were subject to smoke control.

The Alkali and Clean Air Inspectorate is responsible in England, under the Secretary of State for the Environment, for enforcing control of emissions to the air of noxious and offensive substances, including smoke, grit and dust from certain industrial processes.

In addition to the products of combustion already mentioned, petrol gives off exhaust gases containing a high percentage of carbon monoxide. The same gas is discharged from slow combustion furnaces. Carbon monoxide has a stronger affinity for hæmoglobin than oxygen, therefore it is a highly dangerous gas to inhale in large quantities. In normal conditions the amount of this gas present in the atmosphere does not constitute a danger.

Purified gas and diesel oil, when burnt, give off sulphur dioxide in relatively small quantities, but even so add to the pollution of the atmosphere.

Engines of any sort burning petrol or diesel oil give off dense smoke, and pollute the atmosphere if they are dirty or in poor working condition.

(3) **Decomposition of Organic Matter.** Decaying animal and vegetable matter pollute the atmosphere with unpleasant odours, but do not usually constitute a danger. Micro-organisms are seldom transmitted in this way. It must not be thought, however, that exposed organic matter is harmless in other respects.

(4) **Dust.** This pollutes the atmosphere in varying quantities. It consists of small particles of animal and vegetable matter, and some inorganic material. The latter consists of soot and grit, etc., and the organic dust is mainly shed from the skin and mucous surfaces of humans and animals and fragments of vegetable life. Micro-organisms may be present, and some of these may be dangerous. For instance, sputum coughed up from the lungs may contain tubercle bacilli or hæmolytic streptococci. Both these organisms are dangerous, particularly because they can survive when deprived of moisture.

Dust deposited on walls and ceilings with a system of panel heating is converted by the heat to a carbon deposit, which is unsightly. It also creates an unpleasant smell, but is harmless.

For all these reasons, dust is a potential source of danger and an evil to be eliminated. In hospital, every effort is made to prevent dust collecting and to avoid scattering it.

(5) **Industrial Dust,** and fumes from chemical and other works may pollute the atmosphere and in certain conditions may constitute a danger, e.g. inhaled silicon dust produces in time fibrosis of the lung called silicosis, closely resembling tuberculosis. It occurs in miners and workers in slate quarries.

VENTILATION

This is the process by which air in a building or part of a building is removed and replaced by air from outside. It may be brought about by natural forces, mainly the wind, in which case it is described as natural ventilation. If mechanical force of any sort is used to extract air from or force air into a building it is known as mechanical ventilation.

Air in a well-ventilated room is said to be fresh—it smells clean and feels comfortable. This feeling of freshness is due to the physical properties of the air rather than to its chemical composition.

Fresh air has these qualities.

(1) Sufficient cooling power. 18°C is comfortable temperature for an average room.

(2) Ability to absorb moisture from the body.

(3) The right temperature for the time of year.

(4) An adequate rate of movement. (The volume of air entering a room should be three times that of the room per hour.)

(5) Freedom from unpleasant smells.

Air possessing these physical properties is not likely to fall below the normal composition.

Good ventilation aims at supplying fresh air and presupposes sufficient cubic air space for each individual, that is 1,000–1,500 cubic feet, and an ample supply of fresh air of a suitable temperature and humidity.

In an ill-ventilated room the air may

(1) be too still, moist and/or hot;

(2) contain smell, from organic material on the skin and clothes of human beings and animals;

(3) contain a high content of micro-organisms sprayed out from the noses and throats of the occupiers;

(4) contain an excess of combustion products from heating units;

(5) if analysed show a decrease in the oxygen content and increase in the carbon dioxide content, although even in the stuffiest room oxygen is seldom reduced below 20 per cent.

The Effect of Fresh Air. Fresh air has a stimulating effect on the human body. It improves the appetite, ventilates the lungs clears the air passages and enables the brain to function properly. In other words, it gives the individual a sense of well-being. Fresh air minimises the ill-effects of dust and germs and, therefore, reduces the risk of infection. It should be remembered that the value of fresh air is lost if breathing is faulty. Breathing should be deep so that the whole lungs can be properly expanded and ventilated. Good breathing is also related to good habitual posture.

The effect of the air in an ill-ventilated room depends to a large extent on what the individual is accustomed to. One accustomed to fresh air feels sleepy, lethargic and possibly sick and, in extreme cases, may faint. The skin feels hot and damp and the brain works less efficiently. The results of living and working in such conditions can well be poor physique and posture, abnormal fatigue, lethargy and tiredness. All these in turn will result in poor vitality, poor resistance to infection, less mental alertness and efficiency and a reduction output of both physical and mental energy.

Natural Ventilation. This is the process of bringing about sufficient air changes in a room without using mechanical force. Outside air is kept moving by the wind and by changes in temperature. It is purified by the rays of the sun, and washed free of dust particles by the rain. Suitable apertures are provided in the building to allow this outside air to enter. Apertures must also be provided to allow air inside the building to escape. The size, design and position of these apertures is obviously important in controlling the ventilation rate.

Given these structural requirements, natural ventilation depends for its operation on two motive forces, namely the wind and the difference in temperature that usually exists between the air inside and that outside a building. The latter may be described as " *Stack effect* ".

(1) *Wind.*—The movement of wind creates pressure. On the windward side air will be forced into a building through any apertures, attempting to equalise the pressure on both sides of the aperture. On the leeward side of the building the reverse is the case. The pressure outside is less than that inside so inside air tends to pass outside through any apertures that exist. Therefore, the greater the wind speed the greater the rate of air change.

(2) *Difference in Temperature that Exists between the Air Inside a Building and that Outside.*—If the air temperature inside a building is higher than that outside, the warm air tends to rise and will pass through any aperture provided in the upper part of the building. The warm air will be replaced by cooler air entering from the outside, through apertures provided in a lower part of the building. This movement of heated air sets up what are known as *convection currents*. The rate of these convection currents and the resulting ventilation obviously depends on the temperature difference between the inside and outside air, on the height between the inlet and outlet, and the size and design of the aperture. The high temperature created in a heated flue greatly increases the amount of ventilation.

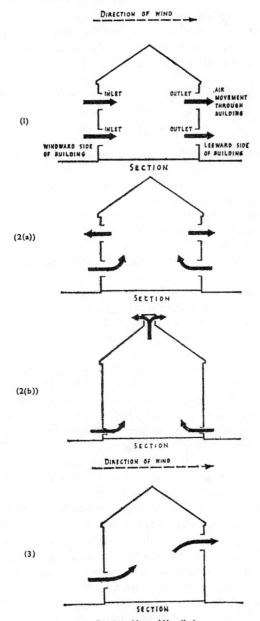

Fig. 26.. Natural Ventilation.

1. Air movement through building due to wind only. 2a and 2b. Air movement through building due to stack effect with no wind, and when inside the temperature is higher than outside temperature. 3. Air movement through building due to wind and stack effect. (Reproduced from *Research Station Digest, No. 34* by permission of the Controller, H.M.S.O.)

In ordinary rooms, windows, doors and fireplaces are the usual apertures through which natural ventilation takes place. Where there is no fireplace some additional form of ventilator is often provided. This is usually in the form of a perforated brick or grating.

Mechanical Ventilation. In large buildings (factories, cinemas, concert halls and multiple stores, etc.), where natural ventilation is inadequate, it is necessary to provide mechanical force to drive air into the building, to extract air from the building or to bring about a combination of both.

Plenum System.—This is the term used to describe the process whereby air is drawn into a building. As it is drawn in it can be conditioned, i.e. warmed, filtered and moistened. Perforated, decorative outlets are usually provided near the top of walls or on the ceilings. The Plenum System can be used to extract air as well as draw it in.

Vacuum System.—As the term suggests this describes a system whereby air is sucked out of a building by the use of powerful fans, again usually placed near the top of the building. Ventilators are provided lower down to allow fresh air to find its own way in. Filters may also be provided to clean the air, and radiators may be placed in front of these air inlets to warm the incoming air. The Vacuum System is especially valuable in extracting unpleasant smells from lavatories, etc.

Extraction units are often used now and are really small scale mechanical ventilators. They are used to extract steam from a kitchen or perhaps from above a steriliser in a hospital ward. The unit consists of an electrically controlled motor which drives a fan to extract steamy air or to draw in fresh air.

The following terms are used in connection with ventilation and should be understood:

(1) Perflation.—The movement of air through an open window.

(2) Aspiration.—The wind blowing over a chimney sucks up the air from below. Obviously this movement is increased if there is a fire in the grate.

(3) Cross Ventilation.—This is the movement of air straight across a room, e.g. through an open window on one side and a door on the other.

(4) Convection.—Warm air becomes lighter and rises. Cool air passes in to take its place.

(5) Draught.—This is a rapid movement of cold air across a room, sufficiently fast and cool to cause discomfort.

(6) Diffusion.—The mixing of masses of air of different temperature and moisture.

Laws About Air Space. In hospitals, schools, factories and such buildings, where large numbers of people live or work, recommendations regarding air space and standards of ventilation are made from time to time, but no fixed regulations have been issued by the Ministry of Health and Social Services.

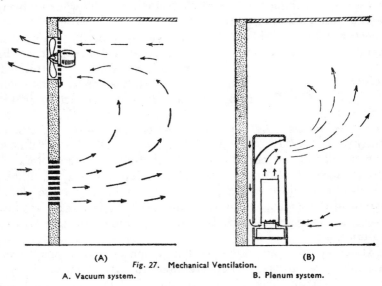

(A)

(B)

Fig. 27. Mechanical Ventilation.

A. Vacuum system.   B. Plenum system.

HEATING

Transmission of Heat. Conduction. Convection and Radiation. Whatever system of heating is used, the phenomena of conduction, convection and radiation are involved. In each case the process is a transference of the energy of motion of the molecules of the hot body to those of the cold; or from a hot to cold part of the same body.

(1) **Conduction** is the method by which heat travels from one solid body to another or along the same body. It is passed from one molecule to another by contact. Some materials conduct heat more readily than others and are said to be good conductors, or to have a high conductivity. All metals, e.g. silver, copper, zinc and iron, are in this category. Materials of lesser density such as wood, linen, wool and paper are poor conductors, so are all liquids and gases. Air is the poorest of them all. Use is made of this knowledge

in the design of cooking utensils; the material forming the pan readily conducts heat, but the handle is covered by a poor conducting material and is often hollow.

(2) **Convection.** This method of heat transference is confined to liquids and gases. Heat is spread by the movement of the heated liquid or gas away from the source of heat in an upward direction, its place being taken by cooler liquid or gas. As long as the heat is maintained a continual movement of the molecules of the liquid and the gas occurs. These movements which are set up are referred to as convection currents.

(3) **Radiation.** Heat travels in rays in the same way as light. A body sufficiently heated to give out light rays will give out heat rays. These rays travel in straight lines and are absorbed by objects they strike. In other words, heat travels from one hot solid body to a cold one, without heating the intervening space. Heat rays can be reflected or concentrated, in the latter case even to the extent of causing a fire. The sun, open coal and wood fires and electric fires are the best examples of sources of radiated heat. Radiated heat loses its intensity with distance.

Methods of Heating. Advantages and Disadvantages of Separate Heating Units as used in private houses. *The open fire* has much to commend it. In spite of some disadvantages it is the most pleasant to sit by and helpful with regard to ventilation. The modern, well-constructed fireplace is very different from the older type, both in appearance and effect. The main points in the construction are that the back is built of fireclay in a forward-sloping position, the chimney is narrow, and the front of the fireplace is open and wide. An inside wall is usually chosen for the position of the fire to make the most use of the heat which is passed by conduction through the walls. Various adaptations can be made to the simple fireplace described. An adjustable air control may be fitted to regulate the rate of burning. In addition, a flap or shutter can be fitted to close the front of the fire to keep it burning low, perhaps to last all night. A boiler can be fitted to the back of the fireplace to provide hot water for domestic use.

As compared with the old type of fireplace, not nearly so much of the heat passes up the chimney. It was considered that as much as 75 per cent. of the heat was formerly lost in this way. Nowadays, much more usable heat is produced from much less fuel.

The type of fuel used varies. These open grates will burn anything—wood, household coal, coke, anthracite, etc.—but it must be remembered that one should make every attempt to minimise the amount of smoke added to the atmosphere. This applies especially to cities where fog is more common than elsewhere.

The disadvantages are obvious. Open fires require a certain amount of domestic labour and will inevitably add dust to the room. If not well-constructed they may smoke and they are expensive to maintain. In country districts wood may be cheap, but in the cities

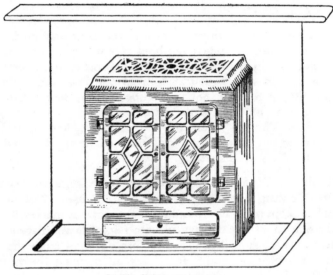

Fig. 28. Slow combustion stove.

and towns the cost of fuel of any sort is high, mainly because of the cost of transport and labour. Also, unless smokeless fuels are used, open fires are responsible for polluting the outside atmosphere.

It is very important to remember that every year a number of people die, or are severely injured, by falling on an open fire or getting clothes alight. These casualties are mainly among the very young or the very old, or those subject to fits of some kind. Sometimes they are among careless adults as well. Many materials used for clothing are highly inflammable and, for this reason, great care should be exercised and suitable fixed guards used in front of any fire where young or old people are likely to be (see p. 125).

The convector open fire is similar to that already described, but is built with air vents which allow cool air to enter behind the fire.

This is passed by convection to an outlet placed at a convenient point above the fire so that warm air is passed into the room. If suitable ducts and vents are provided, warm air may be passed to other parts of the house, e.g. the room above.

Open fires warm the occupants and contents of the room mainly by radiation. The air is circulated by convection, and heated by radiation and by contact with the walls and furniture. If coal or wood is used the chimney should be swept often: if smokeless fuels are used it needs less attention.

Closed Slow Combustion Fires. These are separate closed units, used generally in entrance halls, dining-rooms and sometimes in living-rooms. They are fitted in front of chimney openings. They burn smokeless fuels and, if the air inlets and outlets are properly adjusted, will burn slowly. They are fitted with doors containing fire-resisting transparent windows, so that they have a bright appearance. The doors can be opened if it is desired to sit in front of an open fire. A raking arm is sometimes provided to keep the fire free of clinker and dust.

Gas Fires.—These may be fitted in front of the chimney opening and set attractively in tiled or coloured surrounds. A gas fire consists of a number of gas jets opening at the base of a fireclay back. The gas is ignited and heats the fireclay. The method of heat transference is by radiation and convection, as described for the open fire. Provided they are kept in good condition they are quiet, clean, effective, labour saving and convenient. Connected to a flue they help the ventilation. They are comparatively economical if carefully used. Portable, flueless gas fires are often used but attention should be directed to ensuring sufficient ventilation.

As do open fires they constitute a danger, and should be adequately guarded. There is the extra danger of the gas tap being turned on by children, or left on by mistake by elderly people.

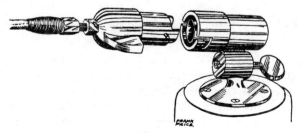

Fig. 29. Safety gas tap.

Special taps can be obtained as an extra safeguard.* It should also be remembered that where gas is supplied through a coin meter, dangerous accidents can occur if a fire is allowed to go out when the gas runs out, and the supply is not turned off by the switch controlling the single unit. Sometimes a gas poker is provided to give easy ignition for an open fire. The same dangers exist with these pokers, and children and old people should be safeguarded from them.

Electric Fires.—These may be fitted against the wall without a flue,

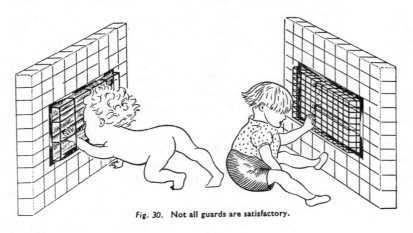

Fig. 30.   Not all guards are satisfactory.

or they may be portable. They are especially quiet, clean, convenient, effective and labour saving, but can be exceedingly dangerous if not protected by a fitted guard. If there is no flue and electricity provides the only heating, then ventilation needs careful attention. Any reflecting surfaces should be kept highly polished and free from dust.

Electric fires in a bathroom should be placed and fitted most carefully, *and should on no account be handled or switched on and off from the bath.* From time to time serious accidents have been caused in this way.

Paraffin Oil Heaters.—These can be portable and very effective. The oil is drawn by a wick from a reservoir; it is vaporized by the heat and burns with a clear blue flame. It heats mainly by convection. Oil heaters are inclined to smell. To minimise this the wick should be kept very clean and the lamp never allowed to burn dry. It should be placed in a safe position where it is not likely to be knocked over, and should never be carried from one place to another while alight. Most especially, *a lighted oil lamp should never be carried up or down stairs, and should never be placed in a draught.*

All the various heating units described above provide heating in individual rooms and halls of private houses, the vast majority of which have no other form of heating. The temperature of upstairs sleeping rooms and corridors should be approximately 10–13°C to be comfortable, a living-room 15–18°C. In the United Kingdom houses

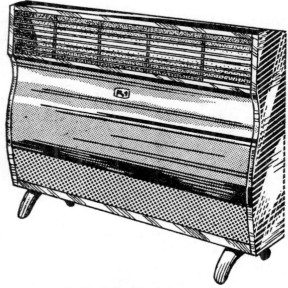

Fig. 31. Modern Electric Convector Fire.

are notoriously cold, and in general, building design does not cater for prolonged cold winters or very hot summers. In the event of a freeze-up water pipes burst and heating is expensive. Visitors to this country cannot get used to, nor understand, our cold houses. Architects of modern buildings recommend insulation of all outside walls, floors and roofs, to prevent heat loss. Some insulation is provided by an air space which is now compulsory in all new dwellings. This insulation may be complimented by lining this space with wood, wool or similar insulating material. This adds to the building expense.

Background heating, although by many considered essential, is still a luxury. The ordinary private dwelling house built by a Local Authority does not provide any form of background heating. Modern units can provide hot air or hot water systems, which as well as supplying hot water will also heat radiators in the rooms and hall, and bathroom towel rails.

With central heating it is recommended that heating arrangements should provide for the maintenance of a temperature up to 17°C above the outside temperature. This will only be possible, however, if the ventilation rate is limited to that for which the engineer has made allowance. In hospitals this is generally three changes per hour.

NATURAL AND ARTIFICIAL LIGHTING

Sources of Light. In the previous section it was mentioned that heat sometimes travels in the same way as light. Light rays travel from the source—the sun, moon and the stars—through space without the necessity for any material medium. Heat and light rays are only small parts of the great range of waves in the ether, all of which are electromagnetic in character. All these waves, which include also X-rays, ultra-violet and wireless waves, travel with the same speed, but differ in the frequency of vibrations and the disturbance they propagate. According to wavelengths and the effect these have on different forms of matter, electromagnetic waves are classified, but in this section we are only concerned with light rays.

The Visible Spectrum.—The source of all natural light is solar radiation, but light can also be produced artificially by heating a body to incandescence, i.e. sufficiently to make it glow. The more intense the heat the brighter the light emitted. Light rays are detected by the retina of the eye, which can aptly be described as the spread-out end of the optic nerve. It can also be detected artificially by a photographic plate. Light rays in themselves are invisible, those in the " visible " spectrum being made " visible " by reflection off material objects. Light travels in straight lines at about 186,000 miles per second. The medium through which it travels may be quite clear and pass light freely, when it is described as transparent. Alternatively it may be translucent, capable of passing some light but not sufficient to render the outline of the object distinctly visible. Most substances are opaque or incapable of passing light rays.

Daylight is produced by the sun and consists of the seven visible colours of the spectrum. If all these coloured rays are viewed through space with none absorbed, the appearance is white. If on the other hand, all the colours are absorbed by an object we say the object is black. Different materials absorb different colours of the spectrum; those not absorbed are reflected back to the retina, and so the material appears to be green or red, etc. When white daylight is split into the seven colours of the spectrum by the sun shining on or through a rain cloud, a rainbow is seen in which all seven colours can be distinguished—red, orange, yellow, green, blue, indigo and violet.

When light strikes a surface part of it is reflected, part penetrates the surface, and part is scattered. Obviously, the provision of good reflecting surfaces is important in making the most of the available light. A smooth polished surface such as a mirror, or a highly polished sheet of metal reflects most of the light.

Natural Lighting. In this country the ultra-violet light rays in natural daylight are never strong enough to harm the eyes. In modern private houses all rooms should be well supplied with window space, which should amount to not less than about one-third of the total wall space. The windows should be kept clean, and curtains of a kind that can be completely drawn back to expose the whole window during daylight. Daylight reveals dust and dirt in corners and crevices, and discourages the growth of micro-organisms. The windows should be opened whenever possible to admit ultra-violet rays which help to kill micro-organisms.

In hospitals of all kinds large window space is provided to get as much natural light as possible. Vita glass is often used to allow the penetration of ultra-violet rays, but it must be remembered that some form of shading is usually necessary in midsummer to protect patients from the effect of too much direct sunlight, and to prevent the ward from becoming too hot. Because, during the winter, it is often difficult to prevent excessive heat loss through such a large glass surface, sufficient heating must be provided to compensate for it. In modern buildings architects make use of the knowledge that shiny surfaces and light shiny paint greatly increases the effect of natural lighting, so it is rare nowadays to see dark brown or dark green paint used in either hospitals or private houses. In private houses windows should not be blocked with heavy furniture, but left clear and accessible. It should be remembered however that windows with wide sills, opening on to a balcony or placed low in the wall, may constitute a grave danger to young children and in their presence should be adequately guarded in a way that does not interfere with the entrance of light and fresh air.

Artificial Lighting. Artificial lighting of some sort is necessary in all inhabited places. It has the advantages of being relatively safe, clean, quiet and labour saving, and capable of being regulated, and is generally most effective. Like most other highly convenient services it is expensive.

Sources of Artificial Light. *The Candle.*—Up to the middle of

the nineteenth century the candle was the main source of artificial light. By present standards its illuminating power is poor. It vitiates the air a little and can be very dangerous. Nowadays it is used for decorative purposes and may be kept for emergencies, but should always be used with extreme care to prevent fire. When gas superseded the candle it became necessary to fix some sort of standard by which illuminating power could be measured, and it was natural to choose the candle as a basis for this purpose. This measurement is still used to-day. A foot-candle is defined as: " Intensity of illumination on any point of a surface distant 1 foot from a one candle-power source, the light being incident normally on, i.e. at right angles to, the surface."

Oil Lamps.—These were used for many years, and might still be used in districts where gas and electricity are not available. They were developed from the earlier crude method of burning a wick immersed in oil. Modern oil lamps are relatively safe and effective, if used properly. They have incandescent mantles, and should automatically extinguish themselves if they are tipped over. They should be used with extreme care, and never carried up or down stairs while alight. Pressure oil lamps whose power of illumination is greater, are inclined to be noisy. All oil lamps vitiate the air.

Gas Lighting.—This was introduced during the latter part of the eighteenth century and is still used in some houses. Gas is produced from coal. The most effective is the incandescent type of burner. The light produced is reasonable, but this type of lighting vitiates the air, particularly with carbon monoxide. It is noisy and can be dangerous.

Electricity.—This is now the main source of lighting. The first type of electric lamp used for lighting purposes was the carbon filament vacuum lamp, invented by Swan in 1878. Many improvements have been made since then, and the process of development is by no means finished yet.

WATER SUPPLY
CHEMICAL AND PHYSICAL PROPERTIES OF WATER

Good drinking water is a clear, sparkling, colourless, tasteless liquid, without smell and free from harmful matter, such as chemicals, organic substances, or micro-organisms. The specific gravity of water is expressed as 1·0 because its density at 4°C is 1 gramme per cubic centimeter. This figure is used as the unit for the specific gravity of all other liquids. Thus a liquid twice as heavy (volume for volume) as water would be said to have a specific gravity of 2·0.

Water contracts as it is cooled, as do most other substances, but it starts to expand again when its temperature is reduced below 4°C. Cooled below that it continues to expand until at 0°C it changes to ice with considerable and sudden expansion.

This curious behaviour explains why ice forms on the tops of ponds and lakes, leaving a breathing space for fish just under it, and why water frozen in enclosed spaces bursts pipes and splits rock. Without that breathing space, which serves also to insulate the water below from the cold air above, no fresh water fish would ever survive the winter. It might even be held by those who consider the human race to have evolved from primitive forms of life to have been a decisive factor in the development of life on this planet.

Burst pipes begin to leak when the ice thaws.

Underground water often contains minerals, most of which have been proved to be of value to the body. Two such minerals are iodine and fluorine. Iodine is required by the thyroid gland to produce thyroxin; deficiency of this substance in water tends to cause the thyroid to enlarge. Derbyshire water is particularly known for this, hence the term " Derbyshire neck ". If a pregnant mother is short of iodine she may give birth to a cretin, that is a stunted imbecile child also suffering from thyroid deficiency. Treatment with thyroid extract can cure this if taken in time. To offset this deficiency iodine can be added to water supplies known to be deficient, and it is possible to buy iodised table salt.

Fluorine is the other substance sometimes found to be deficient, and this is believed to be responsible for a certain amount of dental decay. In June 1963, the Minister of Health issued a general approval to local authorities to arrange, in areas where water supplies are naturally deficient in fluoride, for the addition of fluoride to the level appropriate for prevention of dental caries. By 1968 further encouragement was given and by the end of the year one hundred and thirteen local authorities—representing over sixty per cent of the population—had resolved in favour of fluoridation. In spite of this, by the end of 1972 there was still only a small percentage of the total population (around 16 million) receiving this protection.

Reports have shown substantial improvements in dental health of young children in fluoridation areas, with considerable reduction in the decay in permanent teeth of children up to 10 yrs—the oldest at that time to have received fluoridated water since birth. Experience in other parts of the world shows benefit in adult life. New Zealand and Eire have gone forward on a national scale.

REQUIREMENTS OF THE INDIVIDUAL AND THE COMMUNITY

The people of this country have come to expect a constant supply of pure water. In some areas it is not easily provided. Water supplies

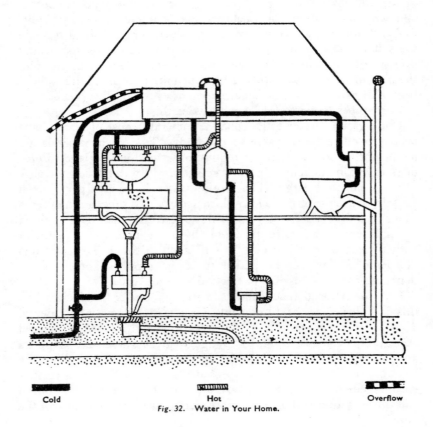

Cold   Hot   Overflow

Fig. 32. Water in Your Home.

were first regulated in the sixteenth century as one of the steps taken to check the spread of plague and other dangerous diseases. The responsibility for national supplies rests with the Ministry for the Environment who depute their powers to Local Authorities. Most water supplies were originally publicly owned. The average person thinks of pure water as bacteriologically and chemically safe, but a chemist's idea of pure water is that which has been distilled and is, therefore, pure compound H_2O.

The overall average amount used per head of the population in this country is somewhere in the region of forty gallons per day. It is rather more than this in the cities and towns because of the number and variety of public services and industries. In certain industrial areas the amount may be as much as one hundred gallons. Waste for any reason, should be prevented. A worn washer causing a leaking tap, or a small hole in a pipe, will cause considerable loss. As much as 300 gallons of water a day may run to waste through a hole as small as $\frac{1}{32}$in. in diameter (the size of a large pinhead). Leaks are detected by turncocks, engineers using special wooden trumpets as doctors use stethoscopes. They set a stethoscope against each service pipe junction and listen to the flow. An excessive flow will be noticed on the meters at the water works or on the meters normally fitted into the water systems of large users such as factories, hospitals, and schools. If no reason for such flow is apparent a leak is indicated.

Water is provided for the following purposes:

(1) *Individual—household and domestic.*—Drinking, cooking and personal washing. Baths: the average bath takes twenty to thirty gallons. Flushing lavatories: the average cistern holds about two to three gallons. Household laundry, washing and cleaning. If a special water rate is paid, water may be used for car washing and watering the garden. In the event of a drought the authority may issue a request for restraint, or may forbid the use of water altogether for these purposes.

(2) *Municipal.*—Local Authorities use a fair amount for cleaning streets and flushing sewers; for public lavatories, baths, swimming pools and fire fighting services. Hospitals, schools and other institutions require a good deal too.

(3) *Trade.*—The amount provided for this varies according to locality.

(4) A small amount of unavoidable waste is always allowed for.

Water supplied through the mains has undergone extensive treat-

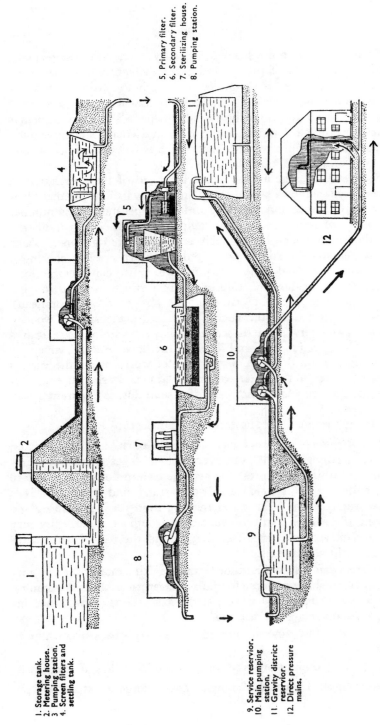

1. Storage tank.
2. Metering house.
3. Pumping station.
4. Screen filters and settling tank.

5. Primary filter.
6. Secondary filter.
7. Sterilizing house.
8. Pumping station.

9. Service reservoir.
10. Main pumping station.
11. Gravity district reservoir.
12. Direct pressure mains.

Fig. 33. Our Water Supply.

ment. Collection, storage, purification and distribution are costly. The cost is borne either by the Local Authority and recovered from consumers through general or special water rates.

Children should be taught from an early age to avoid unnecessary waste. It is now estimated that piped water supplies reach some ninety-eight per cent of all households in England and Wales and ninety-five per cent of rural households and the latter is still increasing.

In April 1974 the primary responsibility in England for water conservation and supply was transferred under the Water Act 1973 to nine regional water authorities, though these may, and do, use existing water undertakings and local authorities as their agents in respect of water supply. At the same time, the water authorities took over the river management functions previously exercised by river authorities.

SOURCES OF SUPPLY

The source of all our supply is, of course, atmospheric moisture. This is formed by the sun's action in evaporating moisture from the sea and from surface water on the land. In the atmosphere clouds are formed and the moisture falls again as dew at night, or as rain, hail, sleet and snow. In most towns and cities rainwater runs away as waste; but in many country districts it may form a very necessary source of supply. The average rainfall of this country is about thirty to thirty-five inches yearly—rather less in East Anglia and rather more in the West country. Rainwater properly collected in country districts is clean and relatively wholesome. It is soft water, and because of this it may have a solvent action on some metals, particularly lead. If it is required for household use it is collected in a well-built, carefully cemented underground tank. In addition, some form of domestic filter may be necessary. Obviously the quantity is apt to vary and particular care should be exercised during the summer months. This type of water is excellent for domestic purposes, but is not pleasant to drink unflavoured.

The rainwater that falls in cities and towns is contaminated with soot, dissolved gases and acids—in fact with any impurities from the atmosphere. The more industrial the area, the more polluted the water. Private house owners and market gardeners may trap this water into an overground or underground tank for household and garden use.

Overground Water.—Rainwater falling on open ground in the country provides our other sources of supply.

Upland Surface Water.—Rain falls on the hills and open land of the country and runs into rivers or natural lakes. In certain geographically suited districts dams are constructed and impounding reservoirs formed to collect the water. The area from which the water is mainly collected is called the catchment area. This area is controlled by the Water Authority concerned, who take steps to see that it is properly protected from harmful pollution. The water from these areas is usually very soft. It may show a brown discolouration from vegetation, and usually has a solvent action on lead. The hills of Scotland, Wales and the Lake District provide large and satisfactory catchment areas. Water from these areas provides the supply for the towns and cities of the Midlands and the North of England. The cotton and textile industries have developed in these areas because of the abundant supply of soft water. The fact that most natural lakes are on high land is a distinct advantage, as gravity is often sufficient to send the flow of water to the districts to be supplied. Artificial lakes are made in upland areas in order to make use of gravity in this way.

Rivers. A good deal of overground water is collected in rivers. A fair amount of underground water also finds its way into rivers through natural springs. Because of its constant movement, exposure of its surface to air and sunlight, and its aquatic and vegetable life, river water in its natural state can be relatively clean. In this country, however, it is rarely so. Most rivers are heavily polluted by centres of population, farm animals and birds. In the past many sewers were allowed to empty directly into the rivers; they still do so indirectly, but more stringent rules are in force now to render the effluent relatively safe. In addition, all river water used for domestic purposes is carefully purified. At the present time considerable concern is expressed about pollution of rivers by trade waste and detergents. Not only is it unsightly but fish life is poisoned and spawning and breeding beds are damaged. The water authorities exercise control over the prevention of river pollution.—See page 161.

Like other overground water, most river water is soft. Some contains minerals from deep springs. The supply is abundant but because of heavy contamination thorough purification is necessary before it is fit to distribute for household use. Most of London's population uses water drawn from the Thames.

Small Natural Lakes, Ponds and Streams. In the past some remote village populations have had to rely on these for their supplies of water. A few still do, and are in difficulty during long summer seasons, when they often dry up completely. When this happens, water has to be transported in water carts from the nearest source of supply. Their water is most unreliable in quality also, and should never be used for drinking without first being boiled. Farmers use it for farm purposes and animal feeding, but it may not be used for washing milk containers, etc., unless it has first been sterilised.

Underground Water. Much of the rainfall percolates through the earth to become subsoil water in shallow springs and wells.

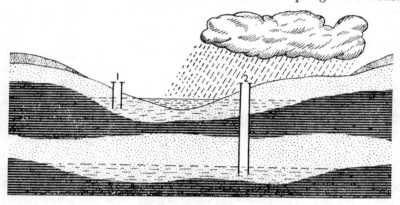

1. Shallow well tapping water from first PERVIOUS layer. Water liable to contaminations.
2. Deep well tapping water from below first IMPERVIOUS layer. If well properly constructed water should be safe.

Fig. 34. Underground Water.

Some collects beneath the impervious layers of rock in deep water supplies. This deep water may come naturally to the surface from deep springs, or may form large underground lakes which can be tapped to produce artesian wells. How deeply this water percolates and in what direction it flows depends on the geological formation. The earth's crust is formed of layers of pervious and impervious material. The former is soft and allows the water to drain through, the latter is hard and resists the water, unless it is fissured or otherwise damaged.

Generally speaking, subsoil water is reasonably soft. As a source of supply it is unreliable in both quality and quantity. If the surface soil through which the water percolates is healthy and well drained, a certain amount of natural purification will take place, but this is not sufficiently reliable to be safe. In any case, the water can so easily be contaminated by surface manure. Quantity is apt to be

seriously diminished during the summer months. Subsoil or surface springs occur when the first impervious strata comes naturally
near the surface. The flow of water may be constant or intermittent.
A shallow well is formed by tapping the subsoil water.

Deep Water. In contrast to subsoil water, that which has collected
below one or more impervious layers is relatively pure, but owing
to the amount of calcium and magnesium salts it has dissolved, it is
usually hard. As a rule the supply is reliable; having travelled some
distance and collected over a long period it is not much affected by
immediate rainfall. Deep water comes to the surface naturally, as
does the subsoil water, in the form of deep springs and wells, or it
may be brought to the surface by artificial means. Although it is
true that deep water is relatively pure, it must not be thought absolutely
safe from contamination. Pollution can occur if there is a fault in
the impervious layer above the water, it or may be polluted at the
exit. The lining of the well may be at fault, or the mouth of a
deep spring may be contaminated.

Deep Spring. This occurs where a second or deeper impervious
layer comes naturally to the surface. The water flow may be constant
or intermittent. It can prove a useful source if the water is properly
collected. Sometimes a deep spring will be found where there is a
fault in the impervious layer above an underground supply of water.
The pressure may be sufficient to force a stream up through the
ground to form what may be described as a natural artesian
spring or well. If this water has dissolved particular salts and gases
it may form a so-called medicinal spring. Such springs are found
in this country, e.g. at Bristol, Bath and Leamington.

A deep well is formed by tapping below the first impervious layer.
Some form of mechanical apparatus is necessary to bring the water
to the surface. An artesian well is a form of deep well that is tapped
in the same way, but the water is usually below several impervious
layers. Once a bore-hole has penetrated to below the water level
there is often sufficient pressure to force it to the surface. The City
of London draws some of it water from such wells.

As the world population expands and the emerging countries
become more sophisticated, the demand for water increases. In
all countries serious thought and much money is being directed
toward conserving the natural supplies. In Great Britain recent
developments suggest that efforts will be made to find economic
ways of removing salt from sea water to render it suitable for agricultural and drinking purposes.

POINTS OF IMPORTANCE IN WELL CONSTRUCTION

(1) The well must be constructed at least one hundred feet away from any source of pollution, e.g. a cesspool.

(2) The site must be slightly higher than the nearest source of contamination so that the natural flow of ground water is directed away from the well.

(3) The well should have a watertight lining which extends, if possible, to below the water level. This lining should be extended to form a coping which rises two to three feet above ground level. Any space between the lining and the earth should be filled in with concrete.

(4) From the extended coping, a concrete or impervious platform should slope away from the well in all directions. On this platform the pump should be erected and the whole area should be railed off.

(5) If a pump is provided it is best placed just to the side of the well and provision made for waste water to be conducted into a suitable drain.

Different methods are used to bring the water to the surface. For a shallow well a simple suction pump may be sufficient, but for a deeper well a more elaborate pump is necessary.

Sea Water.—Because of the inability of the kidneys to excrete excessive quantities of salt, sea water is not suitable for drinking. In the past, it has been used on sea-going vessels and is still used as an auxiliary supply. Distilling apparatus is used to convert the sea water to steam and then condense the steam, so getting rid of the salt. Distilled water tastes flat and needs aerating to make it palatable. It also dissolves lead, so should not be carried through lead pipes.

Quality of Water. *Soft Water.*—Rain or overground water is soft, that is it contains no mineral salts. It dissolves soap readily and does not fur kettles and pipes. It is, therefore, good for domestic purposes. Depending on the locality, rain water may, however, contain dissolved gases and substances from the atmosphere. Soft water dissolves certain metals, particularly lead.

Hard Water.—This is usually underground water. It contains bicarbonates and sulphates of calcium and magnesium. The bicarbonates can be removed very easily by boiling. Carbon dioxide is driven off, and the residual salts are deposited as " fur ". This method is satisfactory for softening small quantities only. Lime is generally used for large-scale softening—this is the principle of

Clark's process. Because this hardness is so easily removed it is often referred to as temporary hardness.

The sulphates cannot be removed so easily. They are unaffected by boiling but can be removed by the addition of soda. Sulphates will, however, crystallise in sustained heat. This property sometimes causes trouble in central heating apparatus if hard water is used without first being softened, and if the boilers are not regularly descaled. Trouble occurs because intense heat is required to penetrate the fur; this causes it to crack, which may result in the boiler bursting. Because this type of hardness is more difficult to remove it has been referred to in the past as permanent hardness.

The Permutit Process may be used for softening water on a large scale or for domestic purposes. A large or small cylinder containing zeolites—silicates of aluminium and sodium—is used to filter the water. Calcium and magnesium are deposited. This deposit must be frequently removed. This is easily done by flushing the filter with a strong solution of common salt.

The addition of sufficient soap will remove both types of hardness. Sometimes the water will contain both types. If this is so, it is probably most economical to add both lime and soda to soften it.

Disadvantages of hard water—it is uneconomic in every way.

Domestically

(1) A lot of soap is required to make a good lather.

(2) Kettles and pipes are furred. This not only spoils them, but is very wasteful of fuel. In heating apparatus more heat is required to heat the water in the boiler and less heat is passed into the room. Boilers need frequent attention to prevent them bursting.

(3) Scum deposits round the baths and basins and may block the " S " trap. This may be a source of infection.

(4) It is not pleasant to use for washing the hair and skin.

(5) It is not good for cooking.

(6) It is bad for washing woollens.

(7) It is thought that certain substances which make water very hard are detrimental to health.

Industrially

(1) It is expensive and unsatisfactory for large-scale heating systems.

(2) It is unsatisfactory for public laundries and for textile and woollen industries. It harms the materials and affects their colours.

PURIFICATION OF DOMESTIC WATER

On a Small Scale

(1) Boiling. Three minutes of boiling will destroy harmful non-sporing organisms. This should be done as a precautionary measure if the source of water is not known to be reliable, or if there is an outbreak of a serious water-borne disease in the locality.

(2) Distillation is useful at sea or in special departments, e.g. dispensaries, but no ordinary household would possess a still.

(3) Filtration. The old types of clay and porcelain filters that were screwed to the taps are now considered obsolete. They were never very satisfactory; they were easily damaged and could give a false sense of security. These filters, known as Berkefeld and Pasteur-Chamberland, have been replaced by two metal types known as the Meta or Stella filters. Both are used with a special type of filter powder, they are screwed on to the taps, are much easier to keep clean and less likely to be broken.

(4) Chemical sterilisation can be used on a small scale—hypochlorite solutions (used in chlorination) are probably the most convenient sterilisers. Whatever is used, great care must be exercised to follow reliable instructions.

On a Large Scale

(1) Reference Should be Made to the Source of Supply

(a) Catchment areas of rivers and lakes should be protected from harmful pollution.

(b) Wells should be properly constructed and protected.

(2) Sedimentation and Natural Purification

Upland surface and river water is collected into natural and artificial lakes. Here it is kept at rest for a period to allow the following processes:

(a) The settlement of all suspended solids.

(b) Exposure of the water to the natural elements—the sun, wind and fresh air, which have cleansing effects.

(c) The activation of a certain amount of plant life. This uses carbon dioxide and liberates oxygen. Too much plant life may be a disadvantage in that it causes an unpleasant taste and smell. It may also block the filter beds. To control the amount of plant life chlorine and copper sulphate may be added.

(d) Natural death of organisms. It is known that organisms such as those producing typhoid and cholera will not survive in stored water longer than seven to twenty-one days.

(e) Bacterial, animal and fish activity. Small organisms feed on bacteria and organic matter. Insect larvæ, etc., feed on these small organisms which are in turn eaten by small fish. Smaller fish are devoured by the larger and, in most cases, fishermen are allowed special licences to catch the fish. All this predatory activity cleanses the water of a lot of undesirable life.

(3) Filtration

After a definite period the water is filtered. As it flows from the reservoirs it is screened to hold back fish and plants, etc. Different methods of filtering are used by various authorities; some use one or all methods depending to some extent on the cleanliness of the water in the storage reservoir.

A Revolving Metal Filter.—This may be used as a preliminary to sand filtration. It consists of a revolving metal drum made of two layers of metal; the inner is more finely perforated than the outer. Water is forced into the centre of the drum and passes through the perforated jacket to be collected and run off from the outside. As the drum revolves a powerful spray of fine jets is forced back into the centre of the drum to keep the filter clear of debris. This debris is collected in a special channel and run away out of the drum to waste. Much of the solid matter that would otherwise flow to the filter beds is extracted and because of this the preliminary filter has proved to give an economic advantage.

Slow Sand Filtration.—Most authorities use this for all types of water. One or more filter beds are used. Each consists of a rectangular concrete-lined tank, about three-quarters filled with large and small stones, gravel and sand. The top layer, of sand, is about two feet thick. Water is piped into the tank above the level of the sand and sprayed in an upward direction. The rate is controlled to give a level of about two to three feet of water, which slowly percolates through all the layers. In about two days a biological green film (of fine plant life and bacteria) is formed on the surface of the sand. This plays a vital part in purifying the water. The filter bed is not considered adequately effective until this layer is fully formed, then it is said to be " ripe ". As this layer gets so thick as to slow down the rate of filtration, it is necessary to stop the water flow, empty the filter of water, scrape off the green layer and wash the sand. The water flow is restarted but the filter is not counted as effective until the green layer is again " ripe ". The period a filter bed will last before it needs cleaning varies a good deal, about two months is average.

Rapid Sand Filtration.—In this the principle is similar, but the tanks are closed and a much greater pressure of water is used, giving a greater rate of filtration. A chemical material forms the vital layer in place of the biological. These beds need regular cleaning. Bubbles of compressed air are forced through the sand and the flow of water is reversed. The extra force used to pass the water through the filter may be that of gravity or it may be mechanically produced. Rapid filters are quick to clean, and are not out of action for so long.

(4) Sterilisation. Filtration removes all suspended matter, sterilisation aims at destroying all remaining pathogenic organisms.

(a) Chlorination.—From the filter beds the water is piped to the chlorination house where it is fed into tanks into which is piped chlorine gas. The gas supply is controlled in proportion to the quantity of water entering the tanks. The small amount used is harmless and tasteless. In the event of bombing, flooding or earthquake causing possible contamination of water supplies, or in the event of an epidemic of enteric disease, more chlorine can be used as a safety measure. This safety measure is also taken when major repairs are being done to sewage pipes. In these cases the water may taste of chlorine but is quite harmless.

(b) Other Methods include the use of ozone, ultra-violet light and catadyn sand, but none of these methods is economically practical on a large scale.

METHODS OF DISTRIBUTION

After the water has been subjected to the final processes of sterilisation, every care is taken to avoid any kind of contamination. The water is led from the closed chlorination house to the storage reservoirs—these also are covered tanks. They are placed at a high level or on special towers so that the water will gravitate to the areas to be supplied.

Water Mains. These are the main pipes which carry the water from the storage reservoirs. They are made of an impervious material such as iron, steel, or concrete. If metal is used it must either be of a non-corrosive type or be varnished. The mains are placed well below the surface of the ground, together with other service pipes, in special channels. Every care is taken to ensure that joints and connections are absolutely watertight. The water mains are the property of the Local Authority or the Water Board.

Street Hydrants. At approximately 200-yard intervals along the mains special valves are placed to allow water to be taken for such purposes as street cleaning and fire-fighting. A yellow tablet beside the pavement with a black " H " and two sets of figures marked on it is the standard sign for the presence of a street hydrant. The top figure is the size of the street main at that point, measured in inches. The lower figure states the distance in feet of the hydrant from the tablet which marks it.

Water Supply—Stop Taps. Somewhere near the entry of the service pipe into the house is placed a stop tap. This tap usually has a fixed tap handle and enables the householder to turn off his supply in an emergency (or when leaving the house unoccupied) without waiting for the water authority to send someone along.

Service Pipes. These are the pipes which convey the water from the mains to the individual premises. The service pipes can lead directly to the taps for immediate use, or into a storage tank which is usually placed beneath the roof. The service pipes are the property and responsibility of the individual owner; they should be laid sufficiently underground to be protected from frost. All plans for the plumbing in any private or public building must be approved by the Local Authority. Where there is a storage tank, there should be one or more taps connected directly to the mains to be used for supply of drinking water. A tap is sometimes placed outside the house for car washing and garden use.

Materials used for service pipes vary; they may be of iron, copper or lead. The latter is particularly useful because it is malleable, but it has the disadvantage of being acted upon by certain types of water. It is possible to treat such water chemically to prevent such reaction. All overground service pipes and water storage tanks should be lagged sufficiently to be protected from severe frost.

It is a good principle to keep water moving to lessen the likelihood of contamination. Therefore a constant supply is provided whenever possible. In some districts, however, it may be necessary at certain times of the year to provide only an intermittent supply. This is necessary when the water in the storage reservoirs falls to a dangerously low level.

CONTAMINATION AND WATER-BORNE DISEASES

Water can be extremely dangerous when it becomes the vehicle for the transmission of disease. During its collection, distribution and use, there are many ways in which it can be contaminated. It is used for many purposes and methods of disease transference are as numerous.

The diseases we are mainly concerned with are those affecting the intestinal tract. The principal sources of contamination are human, animal and bird excreta.

The diseases transmitted are:

(1) The Enteric Diseases.

(a) Typhoid and paratyphoid fever.

(b) Bacillary and amœbic dysentery—the latter is more common abroad than at home in Great Britain.

(c) Cholera—this still occurs abroad but is now uncommon in this country.

Water, to carry these diseases, must contain the specific organisms. They get there by excretal contamination as a result of:

(a) Damaged or faulty sewer or water pipes.

(b) Excreta soaking through the surface soil into subsoil water.

(c) Deep well contamination due to faulty construction and maintenance or personal carelessness.

(d) Contamination of surface water of any sort by infected humans, animals or birds (particularly seagulls).

Water will be the means of transferring these infections if it is:

(a) Consumed without first being sterilised.

(b) Used for washing vegetables that are eaten raw.

(c) Used in the cultivation of vegetables which are eaten raw, e.g. watercress.

(d) Used for the making of ice cream.

(e) Used for shell fish beds—because shellfish are sometimes eaten raw.

(f) Used for washing milk churns or the hands of the milkers.

(2) Intestinal Worms. The ova or embryos of all parasitic worms can be transmitted in the same ways as can enteric disease organisms.

(3) Diarrhœa and Gastric Disturbances are caused by:

(a) Pollution by excreta which contains no specific disease organism.

(b) Pollution by an excessive amount of decaying vegetation:

Upland surface water thus polluted sometimes finds its way into domestic water supplies.

(c) Harmful products of chemical action between some types of soft water and lead pipes.

(4) **Mixed Infections.** Water in swimming baths, rivers or natural lakes used for swimming may also be a means of conveyance of all the above diseases. In addition, it may be contaminated with:

(a) The fungus of *tinea pedis* (athlete's foot).
(b) Organisms from the mucous membranes of the nose, throat and air passages.
(c) Organisms from the skin, particularly of the feet.
(d) Organisms in the urine.
(e) Organisms from the dirt in unwashed bathing clothes.

Because of this danger, water in any swimming bath, whether sea water or fresh, needs constant attention. It usually undergoes careful filtration and chemical treatment. The use of chlorine is usually evident by appearance and smell. As well as being purified, the water is usually conditioned for swimming, i.e. warmed and aerated. At frequent intervals baths are completely emptied and cleaned.

To reduce to minimum the risk of contamination by bathers the following precautions should be taken:

(1) Footbaths of chemically treated water, showers, and adequate convenient toilet and handwashing facilities should be provided by the bath authorities, and their proper use insisted on whenever possible.

(2) Bathers should be required whenever possible to:

(a) Protect long hair with bathing caps.
(b) Use clean costumes and towels (some authorities insist on sterilisation of costumes before their use).
(c) Refrain from using the bath when suffering from infections of the ear, nose, throat, skin or intestines.
(d) Refrain from passing urine in the water. Habitual use of the lavatory before swimming helps to avoid doing so.

(3) Onlookers wearing outdoor shoes should be prohibited from walking round the edge of the pool.

Teachers and young parents taking young children to swim can do much to ensure that those precautions are observed and to train children in good habits.

Ice can also transmit disease. Children should be taught that disease-producing organisms can, and do, survive in ice. It is dangerous to suck ice from any unreliable source, e.g. that which forms on rivers and ponds. Water to be frozen intentionally in refrigerators, should be drawn from the mains, collected in clean containers, and the ice carefully handled, for ice can be infected by dirty fingers just as food.

SANITATION
DISPOSAL OF REFUSE FROM HOUSE AND HOSPITAL

Wherever human beings congregate, they are faced with the problem of the disposal of waste. History suggests that in Classical Greek and Roman times, methods of sewage disposal were quite efficient, but for various reasons sanitation during the Middle Ages was almost non-existent. During mediæval times and right up to the middle of the nineteenth century when cholera was rampant, local authorities spent little on this service. The disposal of waste was the responsibility of the householder. This might have been relatively easy for countrymen, but was very difficult for town and city dwellers. The Public Health Acts of 1875 and 1936 gave each Local Authority the power, and the obligation, to make satisfactory sanitary arrangements for its area.

The methods used for disposal of waste from home and hospital are very similar, the main difference being in the amount involved. Whereas twice-weekly collections of pig waste and dry refuse are adequate for the home, daily collections are necessary in hospital.

Refuse can be divided into two main groups—that which is mainly dry and normally put into dustbins, and that which is liquid and drained away through pipes.

Dry Household Refuse. In both home and hospital galvanised iron or plastic bins should be provided. They should have rims which raise them a few inches from the ground, well-fitting lids and two handles each. They should not be too big for the council men, who collect the waste, to carry. Bins should be kept clean outside and as an additional precaution against rust, raised on two bricks or crossbars of wood. They should be placed well away from any kitchen, larder or nursery window, and at a reasonable distance from the back door. Waste put into the bins consists of dust, ashes, soiled paper, tins,* bottles and other household rubbish. Whatever

*N.B. It is safest to wash and flatten empty food tins before discarding them and to dispose of empty paint tins safely. One case of arsenic poisoning was reported in 1963. Aerosol tins are safer flattened. They may be dangerous if put into a heated furnace with an open front.

is put into the bin should be reasonably dry. Garden waste should not be included. Plastic bags used as bin linings make disposal easier and in some ways more hygienic.

Bins should be emptied at least once a week. In the cities and towns Local Authorities provide for this regular collection. If there is no easy entrance to the back of the house the householder is expected to put his bin in a convenient place for emptying.

Specially designed covered lorries are used for the collection. These covered lorries should have low loading lines to save labour and be fitted with effective sectional covers to avoid the scattering of dust. They should be capable of " tipping " for emptying. The composition of the refuse collected varies considerably with the district, and the season of the year. It is a big problem for the Local Authority to dispose of this waste. In the past it was common practice to tip it on waste ground. This was highly unsatisfactory, as it provided a grossly insanitary area and made the land unfit for building for a considerable time.

At the present time the following methods of disposal are recognised :

(1) *Controlled Tipping.*—Providing this is carefully supervised it is satisfactory. Craters, excavations and waste land can be used. The rubbish is tipped each day on dry land and covered with a layer of soil. Precautions are taken to prevent scattering of waste during the process. Decomposition occurs under the layer of soil and organic matter disappears within a reasonable time. The ground can then be used for agricultural purposes.

(2) *Tipping in the Sea* is a recognised method, but one rarely practicable. It must be tipped well beyond the ebb of the tide so that no waste flows back, and the problems of collection and conveyance are too numerous to be worth while.

(3) *Pulverisation* is possible, and it is known that when all inorganic and organic matter is pulverised it is unattractive to flies and rats. It is also incombustible and provides a useful mixture for fertilising and lightening heavy soil. It is sometimes used as a preliminary to controlled tipping.

(4) *Incineration.*—This is a satisfactory and much used method of disposal. It is necessary to provide a forced draught and to prevent noxious gases and smoke from polluting the atmosphere. Resulting clinker can be used in the making of roads, concrete blocks and filter beds. The heat generated can be utilised to create steam for other purposes.

(5) *Separation and Salvage Process.*—During the last war it was

necessary to salvage all kinds of raw materials. As this was found to be an economic advantage it has been continued by many authorities. For large quantities, mechanical sorters are necessary. Dust is first extracted and used for lightening heavy soil, or disposed of on any suitable and convenient land. Metals are removed magnetically and baled and sold as scrap. Bones can be salvaged and sold for glue making. Bottles can be salvaged, but textiles are seldom worth the cost of the cleansing and sterilising required. The remaining waste is automatically fed into incinerators to be burnt, pulverised, or control tipped. The machinery required for this type of sorting is expensive and obviously suitable only for authorities with large amounts of waste. It is usually worked out on a costing basis and is not done unless it is financially worth while.

(6) *Composting or Decomposition Method.*—It is possible by increasing the action of bacteria on organic waste, to reduce it to humus of manurial value. Obviously all bottles, tins, ashes, etc., must be removed first. Many householders with a garden use much of the household waste in the compost heap. Various preparations such as "Compocyllin " can be used to hasten this process.

(7) *The Garchy System* was designed primarily to serve blocks of flats and suitably grouped domestic buildings. Refuse is deposited in a trapped sink and washed by the ordinary waste water down a chute into a collecting chamber, which may be common to several chutes and may serve several blocks of flats. The excess water drains through an overflow pipe, and the refuse is drawn by suction to a hydro extractor at a refuse disposal station. When sufficiently dry it is destroyed in an incinerator. This system originated in France, and is used in particularly large blocks of flats, hotels and hospitals. Installation of such a system is expensive but running costs are low.

Most local authorities have the facility to arrange for collections of large quantities of waste to be deposited in special containers and removed for disposal by special conveyance.

Waste Paper. Most urban authorities organise the collection and salvage of waste paper. It can be sold to make wood pulp, but unfortunately the cost of salvage often outweighs its value.

Pig Waste. During the 1939–45 war all food waste was valuable, therefore every effort was made to salvage it. Special bins were provided and regular collections made. Some authorities continue with this scheme, they provide the bins which the householder is expected to keep clean, and arrange for regular collections. The waste is sieved and sterilised and used for feeding pigs. All food waste can be used, but great care should be taken to avoid egg shells, orange and banana skins and similar things from being included. Local authorities sell the food waste or use it on their own farms.

Disposable waste that is best omitted from domestic dustbins includes sanitary pads, dressings, etc. This waste is best burnt by the householder, or if no fire is available they should be wrapped in a plastic bag before disposal.

The disposal of waste from hospital is in principle the same, but one or two differences exist. Dressings form a large part of waste which must be collected in the ward and theatre in proper receptacles with well-fitting lids. These are often lined with strong waterproof paper and plastic containers and should be emptied daily. Dressings are burnt by incineration on the hospital premises. Great care should be taken not to put bottles or other breakables in with dressings, for they can be very dangerous to workmen servicing the incinerators. Empty pressure cans, such as aerosol, can be extremely dangerous unless flattened. Also, care is needed to keep instruments separate from dressings. They are so easily lost if put into the same bowl as soiled dressings. Very noxious dressings and plasters should be removed to the incinerator and burnt immediately.

Food waste in hospital can be collected and used for pig food, but special care should be exercised not to put anything in the bin that would be harmful to pigs. Food, for instance, from patients with infectious diseases should be wrapped up separately in newspaper and put in a bin to be burnt. The dressing bin would be suitable. Waste of any sort, dust, food and ordinary rubbish from patients receiving *radiotherapy* must be specially collected and specially dealt with. It is usual for the superintendent of each radiotherapy department to issue special instructions. Whatever method is used it is important to render radioactive waste harmless before disposal.

DISPOSAL OF EXCRETA

Conservancy. Excretal waste consists of faeces and urine. In modern sewage systems it is disposed of along with other liquid waste from factories, houses, shops, etc. The conservancy system, however, deals only with excreta. It is probably simplest to think of this method as a dry one as opposed to that of water carriage which is obviously wet.

On the whole, the conservancy system is dangerous, and in the United Kingdom is almost obsolete. There is always the danger of water and food contamination. The very oldest and most primitive type of " lavatory " was a simple hole in the ground; it may or may not have been lined. It was quite insanitary and is now prohibited by law. The next advance was to a similar construction improved by a galvanised container and a quantity of soil, so that the excreta could be properly covered. If this method is well controlled, decomposition by bacteria is fairly rapid, but the risk of water contamination exists. The bucket requires to be emptied at regular intervals, and the contents are best kept dry. This type of dry closet might still be in use in some remote country districts, but certain by-laws exist in connection with them. The closet building itself must be in a reasonable state of repair and cleanliness and properly ventilated, and the floor must be concrete and sloping away from the structure. A lid must be used to cover the container, earth must be kept available, and the whole structure must be at least forty feet away from any source of water used for drinking or domestic purposes. It must also be at least six feet away from the house. Ashes may be used in place of soil. The bucket type of closet is similar—again ashes or soil being used to cover the excreta.

Chemical Closets were the result of the next advance and have become more important recently because of their usefulness in aircraft, ships and motor coaches. Little space is required. The receptacle is some form of small bucket held inside a portable metal container. A special chemical is used which deodorises, liquifies and sterilises the excreta. The resulting fluid may be disposed of through a simple soakage pit. The chemical repels flies. This type of chemical closet can be used for dwelling houses in remote country districts, but the same regulations apply with regard to the building, etc., as for the pail closet described above. Chemical closets may be portable or permanent. Obviously, the portable type is that used for aircraft and coaches, etc., while a permanent one is useful in a country house or permanent sports ground where it is not possible to have a water carriage system of disposal. A permanent chemical closet requires a tank sunk deep into the ground so that the contents of the bucket will fall into it. A soak-away outlet is provided for the contents of the tank when they have become sufficiently liquified.

Latrines.—When provision is necessary for the disposal of excreta for short periods such as during camp, simple earth latrines can be constructed. A deep hole is dug like a trench, about six to eight feet deep, over which is fitted a wooden box with a shaped seat and a lid to fit the top. Earth is provided to cover the excreta. Organisms in the soil soon render the excreta harmless but it must be kept covered to guard against flies. For obvious reasons, latrines should be placed as far away from the cookhouse and water supply as possible. Cubicles around the latrine are constructed with poles and canvas.

The Deep Bore Latrine may be seen and used abroad, particularly in the tropics. An auger is used to bore a hole deep into the ground about sixteen inches in diameter and eighteen feet deep. Some suitable form of superstructure is arranged over the top. It must have a concrete base, and is fitted with an ordinary latrine seat. Because of the depth of the hole, the excreta does not attract flies and is disposed of slowly by bacterial action and subsoil water.

One of the many problems associated with the conservancy system is the disposal of waste water from the house, i.e., water used for washing and cooking, etc. In country districts this may be distributed over agricultural ground, but there is a danger of the same patch being constantly used, in which case it will inevitably become sodden and unpleasant. It is undesirable to tip such water into a nearby river or stream, therefore some provision should be made for its disposal.

All waste water from the house should first pass through a grease trap or be treated with a special chemical which precipitates the grease, then one of three methods of disposal should be used:

(1) *The degreased waste water is run into a soak-away* which consists of a deep hole fitted with clinker and ashes, etc., covered with earth. After filtering through this clinker the waste runs away to become subsoil water.

(2) *The water can be piped away* to a depth of about three feet through slightly porous pipes which allow the water to escape gradually into the subsoil water. This method is described as sub-irrigation.

(3) *A cess-pool* system can be used as a miniature sewer. This should be well away from the dwelling and at least 100 ft. away from any well. A cess-pool is a large cement-lined waterproof tank, sunk into the ground, fitted with a watertight lid and properly ventilated. It can receive excreta as well as waste water. The Local Authority may provide for the regular emptying of cess-pools, but it is primarily the householder's responsibility and is usually charged for. It is advisable for rain water to be collected separately in tanks or led away into the ground, for few householders wish to pay for rainwater to be taken away.

The Water Carriage System. In this system all liquid wastes and fæcal matter are removed by gravity assisted by the flow of water to the sewage disposal works. It is convenient to consider this system in two parts:

(1) Receptacles and drains necessary for the collection of waste and its conveyance through and from the building to the main sewers. All these receptacles and pipes are the property and responsibility of the house owner.

(2) A sewer for the drainage of waste from a number of properties. Sewers are usually publicly owned and their maintenance is the responsibility of the Local Authority. There are still however some privately owned sewers.

The following terms are used in connection with the water carriage system:

(1) The dual or separate system, which is rarely used now and is unsuitable for cities and towns. Rain and surface water are drained away separately through special sewers which convey it to the sea or river, while the excretal and house waste is drained through sewers to the disposal works. This method is quite unsuitable for cities and towns because road waste becomes so dirty now that it requires a good deal of cleansing before it is fit for discharge into the rivers or sea.

(2) The one-pipe system, as its name implies, is one in which all waste is led directly into one common drainage sewer. There are no air breaks over open gullies and no intercepting traps. The sewers are ventilated by vent pipes. This system is used extensively in America and has recently been allowed in this country. It works satisfactorily in large blocks of offices and flats.

(3) The combined system is that most generally in use in this country. Rain and waste water pass from properties through sets of draining pipes, intercepted at intervals by traps and gullies, into the main sewers where it joins the excretal waste drained from the house by closed sets of pipes.

Whichever system is used, certain basic principles apply.

(1) The construction must be sound and absolutely impervious. It is obviously of major importance to eliminate the danger of leakage from the pipes into the subsoil water wells or into damaged water pipes. The type of construction is bound to vary with the size of the system, whether for a city or a small town. Sewers may be of cast iron, of non-corrosive pipes or of impervious bricks set in concrete. Joints must be absolutely sound and smooth inside. The sewers must be laid deeply enough to escape damage during road repairs and must be made accessible for inspection and repair.

(2) The sewer must be self cleansing. This means that it must be large and sloping enough to promote the flow of water sufficient to carry solids throughout its length. The drains need to be straight, and absolutely smooth internally and all tributaries should enter obliquely in the direction of the main flow. There may be no acute bends to hold back solid matter. Any part of the sewer likely to become obstructed must be made readily accessible—through manholes placed at strategic points.

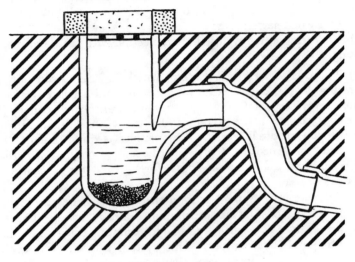

Fig. 35. A Trap or Water Seal (see text).

(3) There must be adequate ventilation. This is necessary to prevent the accumulation of foul air in the drain as well as to avoid the breaking of water seals in the traps by siphonage or air pressure. It is usual to provide vents admitting air at the lowest level of the system, and expelling it at higher levels. The latter usually extend to above the height of the building, and are effective for two reasons, Air passing over the top of these outlet pipes draws air from the pipes. also the sewer gas tends to rise because it is usually warmer than is the outside air. Outlet pipes are about three inches in diameter and the tops should always be protected by wire cages.

All drain openings, other than ventilators and the outlets of all sanitary fittings, should be effectively trapped.

A Trap or Water Seal.—In its simplest form this is a pipe bent back on itself to retain a certain amount of water in the bend. This water prevents the passage of gases from one side of the trap to the other, and is often known as the " seal ". Because of its shape such a trap is often called an " S " bend.

To be satisfactory a trap must be made of hard, smooth, impermeable material, self-cleansing, and have a water seal of depth about

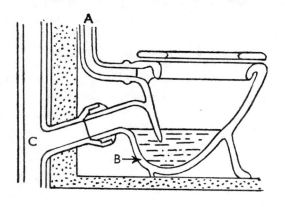

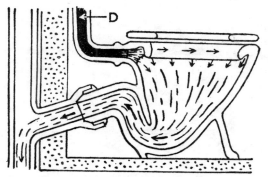

Fig. 36. Modern W.C. of the " Washdown " Type.
A. Flush pipe. B. Water seal. C. Soil pipe. D. Water from the cistern.

two inches. A metal plug is often fitted at the base of the trap if the latter is accessible, for cleansing purposes.

Traps are fitted under all appliances such as baths, sinks, lavatories or sluices; and in the gullies under the open ends of rain and waste water pipes, in which case they are known as gully traps. Intercepting chambers are also trapped. These are fitted in the house drains just before they enter the sewers.

It is important to see that the water seal of lavatory pans is maintained. They may become unsealed by evaporation in very hot weather if not frequently flushed. Periodic flushing is the obvious remedy, but if this is not possible a film of glycerine, added so as to reach both sides of the water seal, will help to prevent evaporation. The seal may also be destroyed by siphonage. For instance, when lavatories are placed one above the other, as in a block of flats, the rush of water down the soil pipe from a higher floor may suck the water from the trap of a lavatory on a lower floor. To prevent this an anti-siphonage pipe is used. This pipe is joined to the outlet of each trap and is either connected to the soil pipe at a point above the highest fitting, or carried up separately as a vent pipe. This pipe is smaller in diameter than the soil pipe to which it is connected.

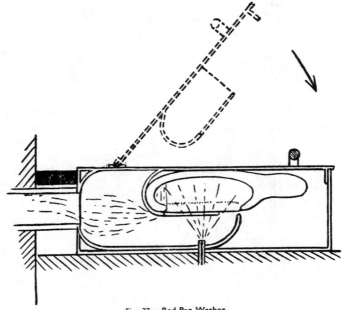

Fig. 37. Bed Pan Washer.

It is useful to have some knowledge of the different parts of the water carriage system, and of the principles of sewage disposal, but detailed knowledge is not necessary.

Sanitary Fittings can be regarded as of two types: (a) soil fittings and (b) waste fittings.

(a) *Soil Fittings—Lavatory Pans and Sluices.*—These are usually made of vitreous china or some form of glazed stoneware, and can be obtained in attractive colours. The trap is in one piece with the pan which should have a good flushing rim, and the whole should be easily accessible for cleansing. The soil pipe leading from the pan should be sufficiently wide. The seat should be well-shaped and polished or washable, perhaps with a lid. The flush of water from the cistern behind or above should be at least two gallons.

The hospital sluice is similar in construction, but shaped to take an upturned bedpan and fitted with a flushing tube for urinals. The enclosed type of stainless steel bedpan washer is obviously better. There must be sufficient force of water to provide a satisfactory flush. Hot and cold water should be supplied, and some form of steam inlet for sterilising is an obvious advantage. The big disadvantages of the type currently in use is the noise created by inserting a bedpan and the weight and clumsiness of the doors. Improvements are being made constantly and disposable linings for bedpans used. Difficulties are encountered when fitting these into old buildings because the piping is not sufficiently large to cope with the extra waste.

The soil fitting is usually placed against an outside wall, the pedestal should not be enclosed, and a sanitary brush in a suitable container should be kept nearby. The lavatory may be fitted in the bathroom or in a separate compartment: in either case there must be a window which provides sufficient ventilation. The floor should be washable, and the walls are preferably light and attractive in colour. Toilet paper should be within reach and the lighting adequate. The latter points are particularly important in lavatories used by children. Paper bags and a Sanibin or incinerator should be provided in any ladies' public toilets and hand washing facilities should be nearby.

(b) *Waste Fittings—Baths and Wash Basins.*—Baths and wash-basins are made in many attractive colours and in varying shapes and sizes and nowadays are often completely built in. They are mostly made of some form of porcelain enamel. All must be trapped, and even if the receptacle is built in, the traps need to be accessible. It is important to have an overflow pipe that can be kept clear. To simplify plumbing arrangements the bathroom is usually against an outside wall. It is important to have sufficient ventilation, and preferable to have washable floor and walls. The windows are usually frosted.

Kitchen and Other Sinks.—The old type of wooden sinks have long been replaced by the earthenware or stainless steel ones with wooden draining boards. These tend to chip and crack and are far from ideal and it seems now time to condemn these in favour of steel (stainless or enamelled) ones. These have the added advantage that one or two sinks can be combined with one or two draining boards, which offers no hiding place for dirt and germs between. The double sink enables clean water rinsing and so does away with the need for tea-cloths providing good drainage facilities are provided. Sink units are obtainable in many attractive colours and may be fitted into a sink unit. The sink unit may be simple, consisting of bracket cupboard and drawers or may be quite elaborate, comprising a refrigerator and washing machine.

The runaway pipe from the sink must be trapped and easily accessible to allow the cleansing plug to be removed. There must be a satisfactory overflow pipe.

Other sinks found in hospital are similarly fitted but adapted in design for particular purposes.

Over Ground Pipes.

(1) *Soil Pipes* carry the excreta and water away from the soil fittings. They are fairly wide pipes with watertight joints, and run straight downwards into the ground. They extend upwards above the level of the house and their tops are open and netted. Any soil pipe must join at an oblique angle and must slope downwards.

(2) *Anti-siphonage Pipes* may be seen led through the walls in an upward direction to open into the soil pipe, or to extend above the level of the roof. They will be seen only on tall buildings where lavatories are placed one above the other. See page 180.

(3) *Waste Water Pipes* collect waste from waste fittings, carry it down the side of the house to deposit it just above or below a gully grating. Again, branch pipes must join obliquely in a downward direction, and main pipes must extend to open above roof level. Open ends need to be protected by wire covers.

(4) *Rain Water Pipes.** —These collect water from the roof via the guttering. Water is usually discharged from the guttering into a funnel-shaped opening; it is then carried down the outside of the house to discharge over or under a gully grating. Some householders collect rain water in an over- or under-ground water tank. The guttering and open ends of the pipes need periodic cleansing, preferably done at the end of the autumn season when the leaves have fallen.

In this country it is usual for all these over ground pipes to be placed outside the house on the back or side wall. In countries where the inhabitants are accustomed to long spells of severely cold weather it is usual for these pipes to be lagged and built into the walls of the building.

* Plastic materials are now more often used for guttering and pipes.

Underground Pipes. All the pipes described above except the anti-siphonage are connected with those underground which are laid in a slightly sloping direction. The soil pipe leads to the house drain which leads to the Inspection Chamber. This pipe is uninterrupted whereas the waste and rain water are interrupted by gullies.

The Inspection Chamber is a manhole in a convenient place near a property and in its grounds. It is covered by a well-fitting and air trapped flat iron lid. The Inside of the manhole is a very simple cement-lined tank. Pipes lead into it on one or two sides and continue across the floor as half-channels, to converge and leave on the other side as one. This one pipe that carries all the waste water and excreta away is still called the house drain and is the property and responsibility of the householder. The open channels and floor of the tank are usually made of glazed earthenware. Although the continual flush of water through these channels should render the whole system reasonably self-cleansing, periodic inspection and disinfection is an advantage. The inspection chamber provides a means of investigation and treatment should any of the pipes become blocked.

The House Drain continues from the inspection chamber, carrying all the excreta and liquid waste from the house in a downward sloping direction, to beyond the bounds of the householder's property and into the main sewer. The house drain must be of sufficient width and must be absolutely water tight. It is usually laid in cement. Immediately before entering the main sewer it is trapped in the intercepting chamber.

The Intercepting Trap and Chamber.—This is similar to the inspection chamber, cement-lined and with a well-fitting flat lid. The house drain passes along its floor and is provided with a trap to prevent the escape of sewer gas back into the drain. Sometimes a " raking arm " is provided should it be necessary to clear the pipe between the intercepting trap and the main sewer. There must also be a ventilating shaft, the open end of which is usually fitted with some form of cover, e.g. Arnott's ventilator.

The Sewer. Modern sewers are constructed to take all forms of household and trade waste. They collect from numerous house drains or small village sewers. Small town sewers sometimes converge to carry their waste to a large sewage disposal works. Small sewers are usually round and made of stoneware or concrete with safe water-tight joints. The larger ones are usually egg-shaped and made of concrete set in cement. These large pipes must be ventilated at frequent intervals to allow the escape of the gas that arises from bacterial action. The open ends of the vents must always be protected, to prevent the entry of animals or birds. Organisms that cause enteric diseases are not airborne, therefore this gas is not infectious. Explosions are, however, likely to occur if it is allowed to collect in any quantity. Liquid leakage from these sewers, particularly during an epidemic of an enteric infection such as typhoid fever, might have serious consequences, for water pipes are often laid in similar channels nearby. Explosions and road mending may fracture both sewers and water pipes. This is one reason why frequent water samples are analysed, and in the event of any risk, or even doubt, the water is heavily chlorinated.

PRINCIPLES OF LARGE-SCALE SEWAGE TREATMENT

Since 1876 it has been an offence to discharge crude sewage into a river or a stream. Since then many practical and scientific means have been used to keep within the law, and in keeping with the tremendous organisation of community life in cities and towns, results have been achieved which are very creditable. The development of mechanised transport, oil from the roads, washings from the surfaces of tarred roads, and the chemical nature of much trade waste have all added to the problem. In spite of it, the authorities controlling sewage disposal are in most cases to be congratulated: one can travel through cities, towns and rural areas, and rarely find sewage disposal to be proving a nuisance, indeed, one rarely sees any evidence of it at all. It is probably the service taken most for granted and the one about which the average person knows least.

We cannot yet afford to be complacent because there are districts even in this country, particularly by the sea, where it can and should be improved, but on the whole we have reason to be proud of the standard reached.

Every generation has its own problems. One of ours is the pollution of rivers—not by sewage but by trade waste. The River Boards are constantly safeguarding the water, having regard to communal health as well as fish and animal life. Much trade waste now is discharged into the main sewers. Since 1936 Local Authorities have been compelled to accept trade waste, but by-laws have been made regulating the conditions under which they do so. The Local Authority has a right to refuse it if it is likely to interfere with the sewage flow and disposal or be detrimental to the pipes and sewers. Oil and petrol are particularly dangerous, being liable not only to cause fire or explosion but also to damage sewage disposal machinery.

For this reason grease, dirt and petrol intercepting traps are provided to clean the washings from works and garage floors, and these must be properly serviced.

Another big problem that seems to have become intensified in recent years is the disposal of storm water. Many sewers are incapable of dealing with it, and improvements are in progress in many cities. In some schemes provision has been made to carry the storm water, which consists of rain and street washings, quite separately, and in country districts this is probably satisfactory, particularly in coastal areas. Most systems, however, are designed to deal with all waste, excreta and household waste, surface water and trade waste. Provision is always made for the overflow of storm water and at present this is being developed. This problem has increased probably because of the increased area of hard surface, both road and buildings.

The Aims of the Sewage Treatment are:

(*a*) To separate inorganic from organic material.

(*b*) To dispose of both by methods not detrimental to the health of the community, that do not pollute rivers, lakes or sea, and do not sour or disfigure land.

Briefly, sewage disposal consists of the following processes:

(1) Preliminary Treatment.

(*a*) *Screening* removes large *insoluble* bodies—sticks, paper, rags, tins, etc.—which are carried away by conveyer belt to be burned or dumped elsewhere.

(*b*) The sewage passes from the screen through special tanks or open channels, through which the rate of flow is reduced so that grit, stones and other small solids settle to the bottom. This solid material is frequently removed, washed, dried and used to lighten heavy soil, or buried in waste ground. The tank is referred to as a detritus or grit tank.

(*c*) *Provision for Storm Water.*—The combined system is adequate to deal with all waste and a certain amount of rain water, but provision is usually made for storm water, the result of very heavy rainfall, to overflow into special reserve tanks.

(*d*) *Sedimentation Tanks* are used after the grit and solids have been removed. The sewage flows into these tanks and remains still for a period sufficient to allow the solid excretal material to settle at the bottom. Chemicals can be used to hasten this process. The fluid is referred to as effluent, the settled solid material as sludge, and the two are dealt with separately.

(2) **Purification.**

The Effluent.—The purpose is to provide conditions which allow an abundance of oxygen to activate millions of micro-organisms. These break down the organic matter into harmless salts, and so render the effluent free from harmful bacteria and fit to be discharged into the sea or river. An older method can still be seen outside small country towns or villages, where the sewage farm is the means of disposal. The effluent is allowed to flow on to designated areas of farmland which " rest " in rotation. A certain type of soil is selected and underground drains carry away the filtered fluid to discharge it into nearby rivers or sea. Vegetables may be grown on the resting soil, i.e. that which is not in current use for irrigation. This method is suitable for small amounts of sewage but would be quite inadequate in large communities.

In large communities two main methods are seen:

(1) *Biological Filtration,* sometimes known as the percolating filter method. The filter beds are large circular tanks four to six inches deep filled with clinker, stones and coke. The effluent is piped to these tanks. A rotating arm distributes a steady flow over the clinker and gelatinous biological film quickly forms over the surface. As the effluent trickles through the filter bed it is rendered harmless by vegetable and insect life. Millions of small flies breed in it, but they do no harm and are rarely found any great distance away. Depending on the nature of the effluent one or more filters may be used. The purified effluent is collected from the base of the tank and conveyed to a humus tank which allows clinker dust and bacterial film to settle. From here the purified effluent is ready for discharge into river or lake. The effluent must satisfy the requirements of local regulations which lay down minimum standards depending on the capacity and velocity of the river.

(2) *The Activated Sludge Method of Purification.*—This is an alternative method of applying the same principle. The screened sewage is led from the detritus tanks to large aeration tanks where the material is allowed to remain for a period whilst it is activated by agitation and bacteria. The agitation may be provided by the pumping of air into the tank or by other mechanical means. After some hours, approximately six to eight, the sewage is run from the aeration tank to a settlement tank, from which the effluent is discharged into a river or lake. The material left behind in the settlement tank is referred to as activated sludge and some of it used to activate more sewage.

(3) The sludge remaining from either method of purification

must be disposed of. It is a mixture of water (80–95 per cent.) and organic and inorganic compounds. It may be:

(a) Dumped at sea.

(b) Dried by machinery or in open air sludge beds, to make manure. If not used for agriculture this can be destroyed in incinerators.

(c) Fermented to produce methane gas for normal domestic or commercial use.

Methods of Emptying Cesspools. Many Local Authorities empty cesspools in their areas. It is done with a suction pump which transfers the contents of pits to a closed receptacle without creating smell or splash. The contents are then taken to the sewage disposal works.

A cesspool, if left unemptied, can become very like a septic tank—a scum forms on the top and bacterial activity underneath putrefies and liquifies the sewage.

Some householders, responsible for the emptying of their own cesspits, use pumps to empty them and dispose of the contents on land by irrigation or digging.

In April 1974 the primary responsibility in England and Wales for sewerage and sewage disposal was transferred under the Water Act 1973 to nine regional water authorities, though these may, and do, use existing water undertakings and local authorities as their agents in respect of sewerage.

Discharge into the Sea. This method is practised in coastal towns. Screened sewage is piped beyond the ebb of the tide; precautions have to be taken by the authorities to ensure that prevailing winds and currents will not drive the sewage landwards. Local conditions must be studied, the possibility of infecting shell-fish layings being always borne in mind.

DISEASES ASSOCIATED WITH UNSATISFACTORY SANITATION

As is explained below, the microbes that cause diseases of the alimentary tract, and of some other organs, are present in the faeces of the patient or the carrier of the disease. Sewage from a community in which these diseases are occurring will therefore contain the causative microbes. If, due to faulty sanitation, sewage contaminates water supplies, for example by draining into a well or penetrating a cracked water main, people who drink the water are liable to develop the disease.

Quite apart from the danger of contaminated water, unsatisfactory sanitation is dangerous in the home or in camps or institutions, since faecal bacteria may be conveyed to people's mouths, by contaminated food, hands, flies etc. and hence cause disease. The principal diseases transmitted in this way, by the so-called "faecal-to-oral routes" are the gastro-intestinal infections, e.g. typhoid and paratyphoid fever, dysentery, and some types of food poisoning. Cholera is also conveyed in this way; though now absent from this country,* cholera is present and indeed increasing in many parts of the world. Some important viral infections, e.g. virus hepatitis and poliomyelitis, are also transmitted by faecal-to-oral routes.

INFECTION
NATURE, SOURCES AND TRANSMISSION

Infection may be regarded as the successful invasion of the body tissues of the host by pathogenic microbes. By successful invasion is meant that micro-organisms, having invaded the tissues, grow and multiply. As a result of this acitvity, poisonous substances called toxins are circulated in the body. These substances affect various organs, interfering with their normal functions, so throwing them out of balance, or as it were " out of ease ", and so the word " disease " is used.

The many factors which influence the success of this invasion will be dealt with later in this chapter, but it is important to realise that infection is the result of a battle between the invading micro-organisms and the tissue cells. The result of this battle depends on the virulence and number of the invading microbes on one hand; and on the resistance of the tissues on the other. For the existence of disease, there must be antagonism between the host and the microbes. If this were not so, one or other would be overwhelmed almost immediately, so that either there would be no evidence of infection at all, or else infection would progress so rapidly that the host would die quickly, probably before any diagnosis could be made. The resistance of the host to infection, i.e. immunity, will be dealt with late in this chapter.

The nature of infection was obscure until van Leeuwenhoek (1675) invented a microscope of sufficient power, and Pasteur (1822-95) began the study of growth and activities of micro-organisms, that there was any real progress in the prevention of disease. Obviously,

* The United Kingdom.

one must understand the source of infection and the habits of the causative organism, before being able to destroy it or interfere with its normal activity sufficiently to bring about its extinction, or to prevent its attack.

MICRO-ORGANISMS. THEIR PROPERTIES AND DISTRIBUTION

Microbes are minute unicellular living organisms. Most microbes of medical importance belong to the Protozoa, the Bacteria and the

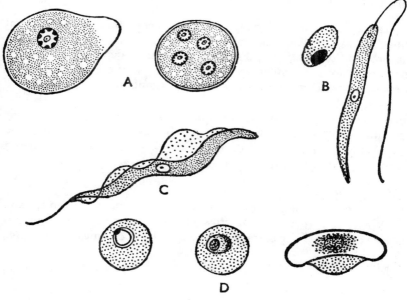

Fig. 38.

A. Amœbic dysentery is caused by the protozoan Entamœba histolytica of which the active and the encysted stages are here shown. B. Leishmania is the parasite of Kala-azar. C. Trypanosomes are the cause of sleeping sickness. D. The stages in the development of the malignant malaria parasite (*plasmodium falciparum*) are shown here.

Viruses, together with a few Fungi. All are far too small to be seen by the unaided eye. The protozoa, bacteria and fungi can be seen through a microscope; most viruses, however are too small even for this.

Protozoa (singular, protozoon) are members of the animal kingdom, such as the malaria parasite, which is transferred by the bite of a mosquito (the intermediate host). Protozoal diseases are chiefly of importance in tropical countries, but some such as toxoplasmosis are world-wide.

Bacteria (singular, bacterium) are minute members of the plant kingdom. They are classified according to their shape, into *cocci* (singular, coccus)—spherical or oval (a coccus may measure about one-fifty-thousandth of a millimetre in diameter), and *bacilli* (singular, bacillus)—rod-shaped bacteria about one hundredth of a millimetre in length and one-thousandth in width; *spirochætes*, which resemble tiny corkscrews, and certain other forms such as *vibrio*. These broad groups are further sub-divided according to their metabolic activities, nutritional requirements and the diseases, if any, which they cause. All bacteria have certain basic requirements which must be satisfied to enable them to live and grow.

(1) **Food.** Protein derivatives, carbon compounds and mineral salts are essential and are obtained from the surroundings, being absorbed in soluble form; if the microbe can be deprived of food, or prevented from assimilating it, it will die. Some antibiotic drugs destroy bacteria by interfering with their assimilation of essential food.

(2) **Water.** Most bacteria die quickly if deprived of moisture, but certain kinds, particularly the tubercle bacillus and sporing bacteria (see below) can withstand drying. This fact must be remembered when methods of preventing the spread of disease are considered.

(3) **Oxygen.** All bacteria require oxygen but vary in their methods of acquiring it. Some, the *Aerobes*, use oxygen from the air;

Others, *Anaerobes*, cannot grow at all in the presence of atmospheric oxygen. They extract their oxygen from chemical compounds in their food.

Many aerobes can also grow with or without free oxygen and are called facultative anaerobes.

(4) **Reaction.** Some bacteria require acid conditions, others alkaline. The bacteria of medical importance flourish best in neutral or slightly alkaline conditions similar to those of human or animal tissues.

(5) **Temperature.** Bacteria vary greatly in the temperature at which they can grow. Those of medical importance like human body temperature (37°C.). Cold rarely damages bacteria, but merely suspends their activities. Thus, bacteria may stay alive in refrigerated foodstuffs, although unable to multiply. Most bacteria are very easily killed by heat—boiling water very quickly destroys all but a few exceptionally heat-resistant forms. These heat-resistant bacteria are

certain bacilli which form *spores*. To be sure of killing sporing bacilli it is necessary to heat them to temperatures higher than boiling point, or to boil them for a long time (from ten minutes to some hours). Bacterial spores are resistant also to disinfectants and to drying. They can indeed survive in very adverse conditions. After remaining dormant for long periods, spores can resume the normal form and behaviour of the bacilli when conditions become more favourable. Thus the spores of pathogenic bacteria, such as those which cause tetanus, can survive in soil and dust for long periods.

Bacteria grow readily if placed in a solution containing the necessary foodstuffs, at a temperature and reaction similar to those of their normal *habitat*. Thus they can be grown or cultured in tubes or dishes of *culture medium*, in the laboratory. The culture medium is an imitation of the solution in which the bacteria usually live. Bacteria of medical importance usually grow well in culture media containing protein derivatives and extracts made from meat at neutral reaction and a temperature of 37°C.

Fungi (singular, fungus) are more complex structures than bacteria. There are many fungi in nature but few cause disease. However, some common diseases such as Ringworm are caused by fungi.

Viruses are much smaller than bacteria and unlike them cannot be seen, even with the most powerful light microscopes available. They can, however, be photographed by means of the *electron microscope*, and in this way clear pictures of even the smallest viruses can be obtained. Viruses vary in size between 0·20 and 0·01 micron, that is, from a tenth to less than a hundredth the size of a bacterium. It is difficult to imagine how small this is, and difficult to imagine how such a small thing can be a living creature. But they are indeed alive, although, being so small, their activities are very restricted. Thus, they can multiply only *inside* the living cells of the host's tissues. In this they differ from most bacteria, which, as we have seen, can multiply if placed in a simple solution of food materials. Not only must viruses have the right food material, but also they must make use of the vital machinery, the enzyme systems, of the host cells. Hence, they can only multiply by penetrating the cells; hence, too, they cannot be cultured like the bacteria, in simple culture media. Cultures can be made only in living tissues. This is now done by inoculating living cells derived from embryos or other animal tissues and growing the viruses in this *tissue culture*.

One fact of great importance is that not all microbes are harmful.

In fact, most are harmless, or even perhaps, beneficial. If it were not for the protozoa and bacteria in cultivated soil, manure heaps, compost, and so on, no higher plants could exist, and hence no animal life either. These organisms cause the putrefaction and breakdown of dead plant and animal remains and render them available for fresh plant growth. The beneficial activities of bacteria are made use in of agriculture, and in some manufacturing processes (e.g. cheese making).

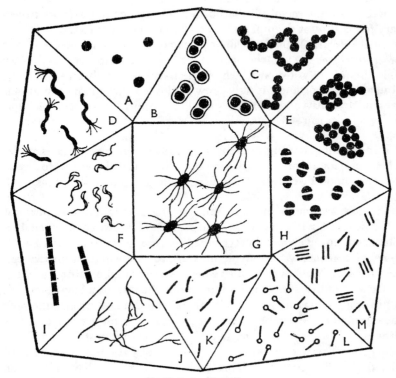

Fig. 39. Various Bacteria.

A. Simple coccus form. B. Pneumococcus. C. Streptococcus. D. Spirillum type. E. Staphylococcus. F. Vibrio of Cholera. G. Typhoid fever. H. Gonococcus. I. Anthrax. J. Streptomyces filaments. K. Bacilli. L. Tetanus Bacilli. M. Diphtheria Bacilli.

Microbes are often classified as *Saprophytes*, which live on dead organic material in soil, compost and so on, and *Parasites*, which live in and on the bodies of higher forms of life. All viruses, as we have seen, are strict parasites; so too are many bacteria and protozoa. But not all parasitic microbes are harmful. Many are quite harmless.

From the day we are born to the day we die, our mouths, intestines and skins are inhabited by a vast population of harmless, *non-pathogenic* microbes. A smaller number of parasitic microbes have, however, the power to damage the tissues of their host. Whether they actually do so depends on the state of balance between the virulence or pathogenicity of the microbes (i.e. their powers of invasion and of producing toxins), and the immunity of the host. These potentially or actually harmful bacteria are the *pathogens* (" disease producers "); although they comprise only a minority of all microbes, they are to us of great importance, being the cause of infectious or microbial disease.

The following are a few examples of pathogens: the protozoa which cause malaria, trypanosomiasis, amæbic dysentery, toxoplasmosis etc.; the bacteria which cause tuberculosis, pneumonia, whooping cough, bacillary dysentery, bacterial food poisoning, typhoid fever, boils. tetanus, etc.; the viruses which cause influenza, common cold, poliomyelitis, measles, mumps, chickenpox, smallpox, infectious hepatitis, etc.

Some pathogenic bacteria cause disease by producing poisonous substances, *exotoxins*, which quickly diffuse away from the bacteria and circulate in the blood stream. Others, the majority, do not produce exotoxins; their bodies contain *endotoxins*, which are more slowly released from the microbes and cause the signs and symptoms of the disease. Some microbes cause disease mainly by invading the tissues widely. Others may invade only to a small degree, but liberate powerful exotoxins which poison the whole body. Thus, in tetanus, the bacilli are confined to a local wound, contaminated with dirt, which is the usual vehicle of the tetanus spores. But the powerful exotoxin, produced by the bacilli, causes the serious and often fatal disease.

MICRO-ORGANISMS IN RELATION TO DISEASE

Whether or not microbes succeed in causing disease depends on many factors, which vary in the same individual from time to time. Most of us, at some time or other, must have inhaled organisms capable of causing pneumonia or tuberculosis, without contracting these diseases. The reason is probably associated with one or more of the following factors. When the organisms entered the body the tissue concerned was healthy and functioning well and was properly nourished with food. The blood contained effective antibodies (see below). The micro-organisms themselves may have been few in number or not very virulent. On the other hand, the organisms even though virulent and numerous, may not have been sufficiently strong to survive the onslaught of all the body defences.

If the body does become diseased as the result of infection by these organisms, it may suffer a mild or severe attack. The body has been unable to resist the organisms and so they have entered and multiplied in the tissues and made their presence felt by the results of their activity, which may be felt locally or throughout the body. The reason why the organisms have triumphed may be because the tissue invaded was damaged by previous injury, or less resistant as the result of some congenital defect. For example, a malformed or damaged heart is much more liable to be infected by bacteria than is a normal heart. A few bacteria enter the blood stream of everyone from time to time (this is called bacteræmia). One common cause of bacteræmia is the extraction of a tooth with an infected root. Normally, such bacteria do no harm because they are quickly destroyed by leucocytes and antibodies in the blood. But if there is congenital heart disease (such as patent ductus arteriosus) or the endocardium (lining) of the heart has been damaged by a previous attack of rheumatic fever, the bacteria may establish themselves and grow on the endocardium causing *bacterial endocarditis*.

Another example of how damage to tissue can lower resistance to infection is provided by the effect of " smog " (fog containing irritant material derived from smoke) which may precipitate an attack of acute bronchitis or broncho-pneumonia by damaging the lining of the bronchi and rendering them susceptible to attack by bacteria from the upper respiratory tract. Excessive smoking may have a similar effect.

There are also other factors for which we have, as yet, no real explanation. Certain micro-organisms, or their toxins, seem to be selective in the tissue they attack, e.g. poliomyelitis virus and tetanus toxin attack the nervous system, influenza virus the bronchi, and lungs, and so on. Also it is strange that some organisms can live without causing any trouble in one part of the body, and yet when transferred to another will cause disease. For instance, Escherichie coli (often called B. coli) normally lives in the large bowel and performs useful work providing it stays there—but if it gets into the urinary tract it may cause cystitis or pyelitis; if it enters the peritoneum it may cause peritonitis.

Another interesting fact is that certain micro-organisms are specific in their action—i.e. they will always cause the same sort of signs and symptoms, will always take about the same time to incubate, and cause a disease that will run a typical course. Measles is an example of a specific infection.

Some microbes have more than one specific effect, behaving in one way in one person and in a different way in another. The virus of chicken-pox usually causes the typical disease that most of us have experienced, but the same virus will affect some people differently, particularly if they are elderly: they will develop shingles and get painful blisters in the skin along the surface track of a nerve. Other pathogens are described as having a non-specific action because their effect varies very widely. The hæmolytic streptococci are typical, since they may cause a simple septic finger, a sore throat, middle ear infection or abscess formation; but several other organisms may also cause one or other of these effects.

When several healthy people are exposed to the same infection, for example in an influenza epidemic, some contract the disease while others, for no obvious reason, escape. The outcome may depend on the number of organisms which enter a person's body. A few may do no harm, but a heavy infection by many organisms is likely to cause disease. Alternatively the outcome may depend on the person's state of immunity, i.e. whether his blood contains a high enough content of antibodies active against the organisms. The more virulent the organisms the fewer are required to cause an infection and the more people are infected, as may be observed in an epidemic due to a virulent strain of influenza virus.

This chapter is concerned with micro-organisms in relation to disease, but it must not be thought that all disease is caused by micro-organisms. The body may be diseased by causes other than infection. It may suffer from nutritional diseases (see section II), from mechanical injury, or from damage by chemicals used in industry. Malignant disease or cancer occurs when, for reasons that are not fully understood, one tissue grows excessively in an uncontrolled way and invades other parts of the body (a neoplasm or new growth). Degenerative diseases of arteries cause damage to organs that they supply (for example, death of heart muscle, known as cardiac infarction is a common result of coronary artery disease). One must not overlook the influence that the nervous system exerts over the functioning of the body, for many diseases are caused or made worse by stress—the so-called psychosomatic diseases, e.g. peptic ulcer, mucous colitis, eczema, asthma, etc.

Advances in medicine and hygiene which have reduced the incidence of nutritional disease and of many (though not all) infectious diseases have so far largely failed to prevent malignant and degenerative diseases.

PREVENTION OF INFECTION AND CONTROL OF EPIDEMICS IN THE COMMUNITY

Methods of preventing infection in the community are based on the knowledge outlined in previous pages, supplemented when necessary by legal regulations. The main aims of these methods of prevention may be to diagnose and then cure or isolate patients who are sources of infection; to diminish the spread of dangerous microbes, by means of good hygiene; or to increase the resistance of the population, by artificial immunisation. The success of such measures is shown by the enormous decline in incidence of many important diseases such as tuberculosis, typhoid fever, diphtheria, poliomyelitis. Other infections (e.g. colds, influenza) are less easy to control for reasons that have been explained.

It is necessary to understand the meaning of terms used in this connection which are summarised below.

Epidemic.—A large number of cases of a particular disease occurring within a short time in a definite area. The local Community Physician usually decides when the incidence of a disease has reached this proportion.

Pandemic.—The prefix " pan " means widespread, so this means that a particular disease has reached widespread proportions, i.e. occurring in large numbers all over the world. Influenza was pandemic after the 1914–18 War, and in 1957–58.

Endemic.—A disease which is always present in one area or country. Typhus used to be endemic in Russia, and in this country and Ireland.

Sporadic.—Scattered or isolated cases.

Quarantine.—The period of time during which it is necessary to keep under observation any person who has been in contact with a disease, in case he has contracted it. It is usually a few days longer than the incubation period for that particular disease. The name is derived from " quaranta," the Italian for forty, because forty days was believed formerly to be the minimum time a ship should be kept under observation after coming from an infected country.

Incubation.—The period which elapses between the entry of

micro-organisms into the body and the onset of signs and symptoms. This period varies with different diseases.

Isolation.—The separation of a person suspected of or actually suffering from an infectious disease from others. The person may be kept in isolation alone or with others suffering from the same disease. The isolation period is the time during which a patient with an infectious disease is considered capable of infecting others.

Barrier Nursing.—A method in which a patient suffering from an infectious disease can be nursed among those not so infected. See page 201.

Fomites (singular, *fomes*).—Inanimate objects which have been in contact with an infectious person and which may, therefore, be contaminated with organisms and so capable of transmitting the same disease (e.g. books, toys, tooth mugs.)

Contagious.—Describes a disease which is spread by direct contact usually by means of infected secretions.

Immunity.—The power possessed by an individual of resisting disease.

Specific Immunity.—The power possessed by an individual to resist a particular disease; may be inborn or acquired. See page 266.

Specific.—Refers to one particular type.

Disease.—Out of ease—any change from normal in the tissues.

Immunisation.—The process of rendering a person immune to a certain disease by injecting him with a serum or vaccine.

Vaccination.—The injection of a microbial vaccine. The first vaccination performed was against smallpox.

Vaccine.—A suspension of dead or attenuated micro-organisms.

Autogenous Vaccine.—One prepared from the patient's own micro-organisms.

Antiseptic.—An agent which is capable of preventing the growth and activity of micro-organisms without necessarily eliminating them entirely.

Disinfectant.—A stronger agent capable of killing some micro-organisms. All disinfectants are obviously antiseptic but antiseptics are not necessarily disinfectants. In practice the distinction between antiseptic and disinfectant is not clear cut.

Sterile.—Completely free from all microbes; the result of sterilisation.

Notification.—The sending of information about a case of infectious disease to the local Medical Officer of Health. Certain diseases are compulsorily notifiable all over the country, others only in some areas.

Infection.—The successful invasion of the tissues by pathogenic micro-organisms.

Pathology.—The study of the changes which take place in the tissues as the results of diseases.

Aetiology.—The study of the causes of diseases.

Diagnosis.—The identification of a disease.

Prognosis.—The forecast of the course and results of a disease.

In practice, the prevention of infection and control of epidemics can be considered under three main headings:

(1) **Prevention; Health Teaching.**

(2) **Notification; Isolation. The Tracing of Contacts.**

(3) **Use of Susceptibility Tests. Vaccination and Immunisation.**

(1) *Prevention—Health Teaching.*—Obviously the best way to avoid the consequences of epidemics and diseases generally is to prevent their occurrence. To this end the government and local authorities appoint officers whose responsibility is to ensure adequate and safe water supplies, clean wholesome food and safe milk. Doctors and nurses, particularly health visitors, teach the safe use and care of these commodities, the value of healthy living, and the protection against disease by various forms of immunisation. Local government officers provide for the collection and disposal of waste, keep streets and open places clean and investigate complaints. Housing authorities work in collaboration with social workers to provide adequate clean, dry housing and to investigate reports of overcrowding.

Port authorities are responsible for the inspection of health certificates of all persons entering the country through sea and airports. If the ship's captain can produce a " Bill of Health " nothing more is required. Cases of smallpox arriving in a port usually create difficulties because we so rarely have them to deal with.

Importation of animals is controlled to prevent them bringing animal diseases into the country. Every dog, for example, entering Britain is required to be held in quarantine for a statutory period of 180 days, the incubation period for rabies.

(2) *Notification. Barrier Nursing or Isolation.*—As soon as an infectious disease is suspected or recognised, it is the duty of the nurse to call in the doctor. On confirming the diagnosis the doctor (if the disease is notifiable) notifies the local Community Physician. He makes arrangements for the proper care of the patient to prevent the spread of the disease. It may be sufficient to arrange for the patient to be nursed at home, but if the disease is serious or if the home conditions are unsuitable he may be admitted for isolation (see page 199) to an infectious disease hospital. The supervising health visitor, district nurse or midwife (now the divisional nursing officer—community) may need to adjust the visits of her nurses to avoid carrying infection to a " clean " home.

If the disease is very serious such as smallpox, elaborate means are used to prevent its spread. Through the medium of the radio, television and the press possible contacts are warned and offered protection by vaccination. The source of infection is investigated and appropriate action taken. From notifications such as these, medical statistics are compiled at the Department of Health and Social Security, to contribute to the general picture of the nation's health.

NOTIFIABLE DISEASES

The law decides whether a disease shall be notifiable.* Each decision is based on current medical knowledge. Any disease can be made notifiable by statute, regulation or resolution of the Local Authority. The last is subject to the consent of the Minister of Health. The responsibility for notifying infectious diseases rests not only on persons in professional attendance but also on the heads of families and near relatives. In practice, it is usually done by the general practitioner, unless the patient is in hospital.

Since 1944 in an effort to obtain more accurate figures, subsequent amendments of diagnosis by the Medical Practitioner, or by the Medical Superintendent of the hospital to which the patient has been admitted, have been invited.

Notification of disease is important for several reasons. It enables health authorities to assess the value of various forms of immunisation, to relate the incidence of deaths and diseases to social conditions, occupations and modes of living. It is instrumental in giving the Local Authority better control over the spread of disease, and makes

* Lassa fever and rabies became notifiable diseases when the Secretary of State for Social Services, and the Secretary of State for Wales signed the necessary Government orders on August 2nd. 1976. Now anyone in the United Kingdom suspected of having contracted these diseases can be ordered into hospital.

it possible to compare the effectiveness of various medical policies and the efficiency of different medical services. Notification helps the research worker to find the causes of diseases, and statistics sometimes disclose hidden relationships between them.

(3) *Use of Susceptibility Tests.*—It is possible to carry out tests on a person's skin to find out if he is susceptible to certain diseases or has suffered from them in the past. The most important of these are tuberculosis and diphtheria.

(1) *Tuberculosis.*—Tuberculin tests are used. Tuberculin is a solution extracted from a culture of tubercle bacilli. Sometimes a " pure protein derivative " of tuberculin, known as P.P.D. is employed instead. If a small amount of tuberculin is injected or rubbed into the skin of a person who is suffering from tuberculosis, or has had it previously, the treated area of skin becomes red and swollen after a day or two. This is a positive tuberculin test and is due to the reaction of the person's cells to the tuberculin, a consequence of his cell-mediated immunity to the disease. A tuberculin-positive person is by no means fully immune, but he is less susceptible to tuberculosis than if he were tuberculin negative.

The tuberculin test is used for one of two reasons—as an aid to diagnosis of an existing infection; and to determine whether a healthy person is a suitable person for immunisation against the disease. If he is tuberculin negative, he is suitable to receive B.C.G. vaccine (see below).

The tuberculin reaction may be performed by

(a) *The Mantoux Test.* This is a progressive intradermal test using in the first instance one unit of old tuberculin. This is injected into the dermis. A positive reaction shows an area of induration of at least 5 sq. mm. with surrounding erythema after from 48–72 hours.

A negative or doubtful result is followed by a second injection of stronger solution of old tuberculin.

If the second and stronger injection produces no positive result the reaction is judged to be negative. A strong injection is not given initially in case the patient is, at that time, undergoing a primary infection.

A positive reaction to these tests shows that the individual has active tuberculosis or has at some time undergone a primary infection and so has developed some immunity. In this case he should have a chest X-ray to eliminate the former. Conversely, a negative reaction suggests the individual has not yet suffered a primary infection, will possibly not have any immunity and, therefore, is a suitable subject for B.C.G. vaccination.

(b) *The Heaf Multiple Puncture tuberculin test.* This tuberculin test claims to provide the utmost standardisation. No syringe is used. A special preparation known as P.P.D. (Weybridge) tuberculin is used. A film of it is placed on the prepared forearm with a sterile platinum loop and a special instrument called Heaf's multiple puncture outfit is used. This causes several minute punctures of the skin, sufficient to allow the P.P.D to enter. No dressing is required, but the area should be allowed to dry for about one minute. The result can be read after 72 hours and may be left for five days. A positive reading is indicated by palpable induration of at least four puncture points.

(c) *The tuberculin jelly patch test* is satisfactory for testing people up to 20 years of age. The skin in a convenient site such as the upper arm or over the sternum is cleaned by acetone or ether. The area to which the jelly is to be applied is stroked lightly six times with " flour paper "—a very fine grade of sandpaper. The jelly is applied in the shape of a V, each limb about one inch long, while the control is applied to the skin just above the V. Adequate cover is provided by a square of adhesive strapping, which must be left dry and undisturbed for 48 hours. After this time the area may be washed and the test is read from 48 to 72 hours from the time of application. A reaction is shown by a V-shaped area of redness and thickening of the skin on which lie small vesicles. At least four vesicles should be present to justify a reading of " positive ". This test is less often used nowadays and is tending to be replaced by (b).

(2) **Diphtheria**—*the Schick Test.* An intradermal injection of a small amount of diphtheria toxin into the forearm causes a round inflamed area if the person has no immunity against the disease. If he is immune his antibodies will neutralise the toxin and there will be no reaction. A person with a positive reaction should be immunised. In practice, the Schick test is not required before immunising young children; they are very unlikely to have acquired immunity naturally.

VACCINATION AND IMMUNISATION

Children should be actively immunised in early life against diphtheria, tetanus, whooping cough, poliomyelitis, smallpox, and perhaps measles. Immunisation against tuberculosis is usually given at 14 years but can be given earlier to children who are likely to be exposed to high risk of infection, and also, later, to nurses and medical students who are tuberculin-negative.

As a result of immunisation, smallpox, diphtheria and poliomyelitis which formerly were common, have become very rare. Tetanus is almost entirely preventable. Vaccination against tuberculosis and typhoid fever though less effective is certainly worthwhile.

The speed of modern travel has increased the danger of introduction into the country of diseases that are normally rare or absent. A traveller by sea, who is incubating smallpox, will probably become ill, and the diagnosis will be made before he arrives. But if he travels by air several days may elapse, after arrival, before he becomes ill. An outbreak of smallpox in 1962, introduced by an air traveller, demonstrated this danger.

In April 1974 the Area Health Authorities took over from the local authority health departments their planned programmes of vaccination and immunisation against diphtheria, measles, rubella (girls only), poliomyelitis, tetanus, tuberculosis and whooping cough. Such protection is given either in family doctors' surgeries, or in health centres or at child health clinics.

Area Health Authorities also make arrangements, in certain circumstances for the vaccination of persons intending to travel abroad and of certain groups at special risk of contracting antrax or rabies* because of their occupation.

Smallpox. A drop of the vaccine, a suspension of living vaccinia virus (p. 265) from infected calves (hence called " calf lymph "), is placed on the skin. A needle is pressed on the skin through the drop, or the skin is lightly scratched without drawing blood. A positive reaction (" take ") consists of a papule at the site, appearing in a few days and followed by a blister and subsequently a scab. Unless the blister forms, the vaccine has not taken and should be repeated.

Primary vaccination is best performed in the 2nd year of life. Good immunity lasts for about 3 years, and partial immunity for much longer.

Diphtheria. Toxoid is used, i.e. toxin rendered non-poisonous, though still antigenic, by treating with formalin. Two injections are given, the first at about 6 months and the second 4 weeks later. In practice, children are often immunised simultaneously against tetanus and whooping cough (pertussis) as well as diphtheria, by injecting a mixture of the three antigens known as *Triple Vaccine.*

Tetanus toxoid is prepared like diphtheria toxoid, but from tetanus toxin.

Pertussis vaccine is a killed suspension of B. pertussis, the bacillus that causes whooping cough.

* See page 208.

A booster dose of diphtheria toxoid should be given at about 5 years, to reinforce the child's immunity when he starts going to school. Booster doses of tetanus toxoid are recommended every few years, and immediately following any wound that might lead to tetanus.

Poliomyelitis. Two forms of vaccine have been used. The first, introduced by Salk in 1953, was a killed suspension of virus that had to be injected. Subsequently, the Sabin vaccine was introduced and now is usually preferred. It is a living but attenuated suspension of all three types of poliomyelitis virus, administered by swallowing, usually on a lump of sugar. Three doses are generally given at monthly intervals.

Tuberculosis. A living attenuated culture of tubercle bacillus is used. It was developed by Calmette and Guérin and hence called Bacille Calmette-Guérin (BCG). It is injected intradermally, but only to tuberculin-negative individuals. (If it were given to a tuber-culin-positive person, the vaccine would provoke an exaggerated and perhaps destructive version of the tuberculin reaction.) A small local lesion appears in a few weeks and heals again after a few months. The tuberculin reaction will be positive if tested about 6 weeks after the injection.

Enteric Fever (Typhoid and Paratyphoid). Two injections of a killed mixture of typhoid and paratyphoid A and B bacilli (T.A.B.) are given. Thereafter, booster doses are recommended at yearly intervals. T.A.B. is not needed for the general population of the U.K. but it should be given to travellers to countries with high risks of infection and to doctors, nurses and other medical workers. A similar type of vaccine is used to protect against *cholera*.

THE RELATIONSHIP BETWEEN THE PREVENTION AND CURE OF DISEASE

It has been said that in the future it might be that " a doctor is paid according to the patients he does not have to treat ". This is not such a stupid suggestion. From the time that scientists learnt to use the microscope and to recognise micro-organisms, much disease has been prevented. It may well be in the not too distant future that most diseases caused by micro-organisms—including viruses—will be preventable either by community or personal health measures, including vaccination, inoculation and chemoprophylaxis.

When a physician meets a case of infectious disease which cannot readily be diagnosed he gives in the first instance symptomatic treatment—i.e. treatment intended to relieve pain and to maintain bodily efficiency. Then he confers with specialists (pathologists, radiologists, etc.) for the purpose of identifying the disease.

Organisms which might be causing the disease are isolated from the patient's body and bred in culture. A study of their modes of breeding and growth can indicate their family groups. Sometimes the toxins also and their effects on the body are studied (toxins are harmful substances produced by the organism).

Known methods of attacking germs are tried on the culture-bred organisms. "Bactericidal" drugs (which kill bacteria), "bacteriostatic" drugs (which make them inactive) and "antibiotics" (culture-bred germicides such as penicillin) are used. Synthetic antibacterial drugs too, e.g. sulphonamides, are sometimes used.

When an effective drug has been found, more experiments are done to determine how to administer it and the size of minimum and maximum doses which can destroy the disease without harming the patient. These biological standardisation tests are carried out on infected animals. However much we might regret our use of animals for this purpose we have to accept it as necessary.

After standardisation the drug is used under the control of the Medical Research Council or its equivalent in other countries until its value and safety have been firmly established. Control is exercised through medical schools, each of which is issued with a limited quantity to be used and reported on in detail. After a satisfactory period of controlled use the drug is released for general use.

Much of the research work involved in the establishment of new drugs is financed by the chemical industry.

When the bacteriologist can recognise an organism and control it he can usually find a means of preventing the disease it causes. We know that living blood reacts to invading organisms by making antibodies against them. We introduce into the body small doses of a germ or its toxin—slightly inactivated—and the body builds up a resistance sufficient to counteract a real attack of the germ later. The blood having once learnt how to make an antibody can quickly increase its supplies in time of need. A "booster dose" of the vaccine or toxoid is often given months later to increase the strength of the antibody. This is the principle behind the whole system of immunisation: to help the body to develop its defence while in a fit and healthy state instead of leaving it to chance.

Now that air travel is commonly used general immunisation is even more important. People can travel from one country to another overnight and from one side of the world to the other in less time than it takes for some of the diseases to develop (the incubation period). This means that the Bill of Health (previously satisfactory for protection of the community from sea travellers) is not sufficient to protect them from air travellers. A serious but small outbreak of smallpox in 1962 emphasised this danger.

By now we have learnt to prevent and cure most serious infectious diseases, although proven methods do not always succeed because of unpredictable complications. But by and large, the diseases we have yet to learn to prevent are those for which we know no definite cause—the malignant diseases, the common cold and all the psychosomatic diseases. A comparison of the list of diagnoses in an acute general ward of a busy hospital of today with one of fifty years ago would tell its own story. Many cases of deformity, paralysis and mental retardation which figured in the latter are today non-existent because we have learnt to prevent difficult labour by having a better understanding of pre-natal care. That is because we have learnt what produces difficult labour: e.g. deformity in the mother due to osteomalacia: rickets—a deficiency disease—easily preventable by giving the right diet—one containing vitamin D— and sunlight.

Belonging much more to the present is the relationship between streptococcal infections and chronic cardiac disease. Because we have learnt how a heart becomes damaged we go back to the very beginning and use chemical drugs to prevent children from developing sore throats. It is gratifying to know that by controlling such an ordinary thing as a sore throat one may be preventing chronic cardiac failure in later life.

To consider a hypothetical case: the radiologist takes a picture and identifies a small foreign body in the bronchus: the technician makes an instrument to reach it with: the chemist provides appropriate anaesthetics: the doctor with the assistance of the nurse removes the foreign body and takes care of the patient during the operation, and restores him to health: a programme of team work which prevents our hypothetical patient from at best chronic bronchitis and bronchiectasis—or at worst lung abscess, septicæmia and death.

Sometimes patients die without known cause. If the doctor cannot sign a certificate stating the cause of death, the law demands that a post-mortem be performed. Even when the doctor does know why a patient has died a post-mortem may still be carried out and prove most helpful. By examination of the body the pathologist might discover why the condition did not respond to treatment as it should have, why the patient developed, e.g., pneumonia and so on. Thus he may be able to teach others how to avoid such accidents. So everyone in the health team should be striving not only to cure diseases but also to find out why they occur in order to prevent them. In a way the British method of National Health Insurance is like that, all pay in taxation every week toward the cost of the work of preventive and promotive health, as well as that of curative medicine.

Similar relationships exist between prevention and cure of mental diseases. An understanding of normal human psychology and behaviour helps a doctor to diagnose and cure mental disease, to recognise new mental disorders and to define them. It helps him also to detect early warning signs of mental disorder, and to give treatment early to prevent breakdown. This is done by helping the patient to realise why he is feeling as he does, and so helping him to get over the difficulty. Prophylactic rest may be all that is required.

In all branches of medicine an understanding of the normal helps us to tackle the abnormal. Thus we need to know how normal kidneys work before we can diagnose and treat diseased ones. The aim of the medical services can thus be summarised:

(a) To study the normal.

(b) To study the signs, symptoms and results of diseases.

(c) To find curative treatments.

(d) To find preventive measures.

It is possible to compare doctors with motor mechanics and patients with engines but only in a very limited way—for people are not machines and doctors and nurses need far more finesse in their approach to patients than mechanics need for their machines.

RABIES

This acute fatal specific virus disease—otherwise known as hydrophobia—has been known to affect animal and man since early Greek and Roman times. The virus is conveyed to man's nervous system through animal and bird saliva. All mammals and birds are susceptible to innoculation but the spread of the disease is almost entirely by dogs. The virus is transmitted by the saliva through a bite or lick but it will not pass through unbroken skin.

During the past twenty years the disease has spread through Europe particularly from central and eastern countries, and it is thought that the fox is the principal reservoir of infection. In Latin America bats appear more responsible and cause losses in cattle breeding areas. Some countries of the world are free from this disease, e.g. Australia and Britain. The latter is constantly on the alert for it and maintains stringent but unpopular rules regarding quarantine of dogs. The incubation period varies from twelve to fifty days and the disease once established runs a short violent course.

The World Health Organisation strives consistently to develop a better rabies vaccine for man and animals and works to improve control of the disease internationally. Any dog suspected of being infected should be chained, given water and kept alive until veterinary help is obtained.

A possibly infected person must also get medical help. If wounded, a tourniquet or ligature should be applied within thirty minutes, and the wound bathed and cauterised. The tourniquet should be applied sufficiently tight to stop the return of blood from the wound area but not to stop the arterial supply. The object of this is to allow the bleeding to flush out any poisonous material that may have been deposited in the wound from the saliva of the animal thus preventing the circulation of poison in the blood stream. Once the disease is established symptomatic treatment can only be palliative. Passive immunisation is effective in potentially infected cases and immunity can be given by innoculation.

DOMICILIARY CARE

The third part of the National Health Act deals with services provided until 1974 by Local Authorities (see page 12). These are, comprehensive and deal with preventive medicine, promotive health, and treatment of disease. Many people are involved, all requiring specialised training. Health Authority officers work in close association with those of the Local Authority and voluntary services and with those who work in hospital. To understand the working of the Health Authority one must know something of the various people and departments it controls.

Domiciliary care is that given to people in their homes. As little as a century ago this was almost unknown as an organised controlled practice. Hospitals were established, but preventive medicine, the district nurse, health visitor, and midwife had not been thought of. In recent years, particularly since the war, this service has grown tremendously; so much so, that now not only urban but also all county and rural areas in the United Kingdom are provided with the services of all three. In some rural areas all three services (nursing, health visiting, midwifery) may be given by one person.

HOME NURSING—OFTEN CALLED DISTRICT NURSING

The Home Nurse. The home nurse is probably the best appreciated of them all, because she gives the most active assistance in time of need. She is prepared to undertake skilled nursing of all age groups in all types of homes under the direction of a doctor.

The story of the development of home nursing is interesting. It began as a voluntary organisation and remained one until the National Health Act came into being.

Until the time of Florence Nightingale, visiting the sick in their homes was the responsibility accepted by the Churches. These services lapsed during the deplorable period of the Dark Ages, and it was Florence Nightingale who revolutionised the nursing service generally. In 1840 Mrs. Fry made efforts to establish a district nursing service in London, but the first really successful service was established by William Rathbone in Liverpool. He was a philanthropist who was so impressed by the efficient care given to his wife by one of Miss Nightingale's nurses that he decided to make available such care to the sick relatives of his work people. Because Miss Nightingale could not spare any more of her nurses a school was set up, attached to Liverpool Royal Infirmary, in 1862. Within four years eighteen trained district nurses were working in Liverpool, their work and training supervised by a committee of ladies who gave their services free.

The service was extended by individual effort to other cities, including London, but it was not until 1887 that district nursing became a national institution. On the occasion of Queen Victoria's Jubilee, Her Majesty was presented with a large sum of money for the women of Great Britain and Northern Ireland. The interest on this fund, amounting to £2,000 per annum, was used for the founding of the Queen Victoria Jubilee Institute for Nurses. The Institute was granted a Royal Charter in 1889, and the training standardised. Further large sums of money were added on the occasion of Her Majesty's Diamond Jubilee. Most of the existing associations had by this time accepted conditions of affiliation.

The organisation grew and prospered steadily, further sums were added to the fund and new training schools started. When Queen Mary succeeded as Patron the name was changed to " The Queen's Institute of District Nursing," the name that is used today. A supplementary Charter was issued in 1928.

The greatest need for these services was understandably in our cities, especially around the poverty ridden dock areas. Patients paid according to their means, and the service was controlled by committees of lay people. Patients who could afford full payment were advised to obtain the services of a private nurse. It was the rule that the district nurse, at the request of the doctor, attended the sick poor, irrespective of race or creed.

On the appointed day when the National Health Act came into force the Local Authorities were given the responsibility for nursing people in their homes. The service was already there, and while in some instances the authorities took over direct control, in others they only accepted financial responsibility. All nursing services and the loan of equipment are free. In most cities there is a twenty-four hour telephone service available.

There is considerable co-operation between all the nursing and social services, and there is a move for more understanding between those working in hospital and those in the home. The General Nursing Council recognise this by including Social Aspects of Disease and Community Nursing in the curriculum of a nurse's general training. The Ministry recognise too the need to give Registered and Enrolled nurses further special training in home nursing schemes to prepare them for nursing people in their own homes.

Until recently just over half—fifty-five per cent—of those working as home nurses had received special training but the present objective is to have a fully trained district nursing service. To this end nationally controlled and recognised centres* and standardised examinations were introduced in 1968 and the service fully integrated into those of the local health authority.

The Council for the training of Health Visitors have approved a few schemes for integrated district nurse/health visitor training.

Home/District Nurse Training

The length of training is *four months*. This is reduced to *three months* for:

(1) State registered nurses who are also state certified midwives or who hold a Diploma of Nursing, a Tutor's Diploma or the Health

* In 1969 there were fifty-five training centres in U.K.

Visitor's Certificate, or

(2) State registered nurses with a minimum of eighteen months of experience in general district nursing, who are recommended by their employing authorities.

Students may be resident or non-resident during training.

A national certificate is awarded for passing the qualifying examination. Each year about 700 nurses study for it. At present there is approximately one home nurse to approximately 7,000 of the population.

The post-registration training is recognised as necessary in order that nurses might understand, from social and preventive points of view, the needs of patients in their homes. A district nurse must have a sense of social responsibility toward the community in general and a desire to help to improve conditions in peoples' homes. To do this effectively she must learn to adapt hospital nursing techniques to home situations. By doing so she can help the family doctor to exercise adequate supervision without his having to make unnecessary demands on hospital places. Much of the home nurses' work concerns the care of patients with chronic and terminal illness, the aged and mentally sick, but she must be prepared also to nurse those with acute illnesses and infectious diseases including tuberculosis. She also learns how to enlist the aid of the patient's relatives by teaching them the rudiments of health education and home nursing: and becomes familiar with the organisations which provide other social services in order to be able to bring them to the aid of her patients.

A few male nurses work in districts in the cities and give valuable service, as also do a few state enrolled nurses.

It is interesting that when to so many people in this country voluntary service appeared to be superseded by State Welfare Services it began to materialise in less developed countries. Many people from all parts of the world come to this country to observe our methods of training and work and Queen's Nurses go out to many parts of the world to help and to train workers in less developed nations.

MATERNITY AND CHILD HEALTH SERVICES

The Area Health Authorities have since 1st April 1974 taken over responsibility for maternity and child health services, including the community health services previously administered by local authorities and the medical and dental inspection and treatment functions of the school health services formerly provided by local education authorities. The community health services include a network of maternity and child health centres, the more recent of which have usually been built as part of all-purpose health centres.

HEALTH VISITING

The Health Visitor. The health visitor is mainly a social adviser and health educator. She aims to encourage and promote full health of mind and body within family groups. She co-operates with other health and social workers to ensure that the best use is made of the statutory and voluntary services available.

Health visiting had its origin in Manchester in 1862. As did most other social services it began as a voluntary movement and gradually developed until now, little more than a hundred years later, it is a highly organised statutory service. In early years the work was concerned mainly with control of infection and infant mortality, and it was not until the Notification of Births Act were passed in 1907 and 1915 that Local Authorities really assumed the responsibility for providing health visitors.

It was not until 1919 that the then newly established Ministry of Health prescribed a special course of training. This was made more comprehensive in 1925, and revised in 1949 to meet the new demands of the National Health Service. At the present time a health visitor is required to be a State Registered General Nurse—S.R.N.—with midwifery experience and a pass in the first part of the examination of the Central Midwives' Board. In addition she must have completed an approved course of instruction and obtained the Health Visitors' Certificate.

Her function can be described as that of a "nurse with special training in health education, child welfare and social work". Hitherto she has specialised chiefly in mothercraft, though some have also visited the homes of sufferers from tuberculosis, mental illness and venereal disease. But under the new service she is friend and adviser to the whole family for her duties are defined by the Health Act as concerned with the care of children, sick persons, expectant and nursing mothers, and with measures to prevent the spread of disease. (Even the family pets are subject to her eagle-eyed scrutiny if they constitute any menace to the health of their owners.) Hitherto, health visitors have worked mainly with doctors in 4,000 infant welfare centres, but the aim is that they should work in much closer liaison with family doctors, and many are already doing so, thus establishing successful working partnerships. In this way the doctor is able to put the health visitor in touch with the families who need her. In order for her to do this, the estimated number of health visitors required is based on the whole population, not as previously on the number of children under 5 years old.

Such an extension of the health visitor's duties has led to an increase in required numbers—from a previous 1 for 6,500 of the population to a future 1 for 4,500.

Health Visitor Training

Training is under the control of the Council for the Training of Health Visitors. There are about thirty-one centres (8–9,000 places) in England providing ordinary post-registration courses and six providing integrated district nurse/health visitor training. These centres are associated with Universities, Polytechnic and Professional Colleges.

The health visitor's duties may be summarised as follows:

A. *The Care of Mothers and Children.*

(1) *The care of expectant mothers.*—She gives advice on everything to do with the mental and physical well-being of mothers as well as preparation for the confinement.

She attends antenatal clinics to explain what the doctor means and to give talks and practical demonstrations to groups of expectant mothers.

(2) *Home visiting.*—She visits homes to give advice about promoting the mental and physical well-being of all members of the family, and to reinforce the stability of the home. She follows up, supervises and reports on the progress of children suffering from illness or physical handicap, and especially children who are illegitimate, or who for any period are cared for away from home. (In this latter respect she works in collaboration with the local authority welfare services. She helps and advises in co-operation with these same services any family presenting a social problem. She investigates the causes of still-births, neonatal and accidental deaths, and helps unmarried mothers to rehabilitate themselves. She co-operates with the hospital medico social case workers in making enquiries and arrangements for admission to and discharge from hospital and helps with arrangements for convalescence and holidays. She plays an active part in the prevention of accidents in the home by continually observing conditions, advising on avoidance of dangers, and investigating the history of all children who have suffered preventable

injuries, particularly burns. She assists generally in the collection of statistics, and co-operates in any research which has a bearing on the welfare of the family as a whole.

(3) *Duties in Maternity and Child Welfare Services.*—She interviews and advises all mothers attending these clinics, assists the doctor as necessary and carries out a programme of health education.

B. Responsibilities Towards the School Health Service.

A school nurse requires the same qualifications as a health visitor. Their duties are part advisory and part teaching; attending all school medical examinations to give the children, parents and doctors any help required; treating the children and advising and helping the parents of any children found to be verminous or suffering minor complaints, or those with any defect or requiring special appliances or occupational training; co-operating with teachers and parents in understanding difficulties and promoting the well-being of the home and family and assisting in any scheme for training in parentcraft, homecraft and citizenship.

C. Prevention of Infectious Disease.

She takes every opportunity of teaching the causes of infection; encourages prevention by explaining measures used to immunise and vaccinate children against it; makes arrangements for the care of those suffering an infectious disease, and advises on disinfection. She assists in all schemes for the control of infection, co-operating with general practitioners and the Community Physician. She is concerned with the personal and clinical aspects, whereas the Public Health Officer deals with insanitary housing and disinfection of premises.

D. Care and After Care.

Illness—of Body or Mind. The National Health Service Act, 1946, requires the health visitor to give advice on the care of persons suffering from illness (which by the definition in Section 79 includes mental illness). The Mental Health Act, 1959, places responsibility on local health authorities to develop community services for the mentally sick.

The health visitor is prepared by her training to recognise deviations from the normal in physical and mental health. In her contact with families she becomes aware of early stress or tensions and can advise them to obtain medical or other aid, or with their permission herself seeks the help of other workers before breakdown occurs.

The Mentally Disordered. A health visitor is often the first person to suspect mental sub-normality in a young child. She encourages parents to seek medical advice and helps them to accept the child's handicap. She gives particulars to the Community Physician in order that services for the care and training of the mentally handicapped may be used at the appropriate time.

She may also have responsibilities with regard to the care and rehabilitation of the mentally ill.

The Elderly. A health visitor's duties include attention to the needs of the elderly either within a family circle or when living alone. She gets to know the elderly in her area through a variety of contacts. She may be able to help the family to adjust and meet their needs, and can encourage solitary elder citizens to make use of community resources and voluntary services. She also co-operates with the general practitioner, district nurse, home help organiser or geriatric team in meeting social needs. She can help to arrange temporary hospital accommodation for an elderly infirm member of a family, to give his relatives a holiday or rest; she can help to promote good neighbourliness by linking those willing to give service with those in need of it.

The care of elder members of the community is a sphere in which general practitioners and health visitors must work closely together if the best service is to be given.

Sexually Transmitted Disease. The health visitor may be required to assist in the follow-up of patients after treatment for sexually transmitted disease and of persons known or believed to be sources of infection.

Research. Local health and welfare authorities are frequently called upon to take part in surveys and research projects, the field work for which is undertaken by health visitors.

E. Health Education.

The health visitor is often expected to take part in teaching programmes arranged for various groups of students undergoing recognised courses in the care of children. She may be expected also to talk to organised groups such as women's institutes and youth clubs. She should be the expert, educating the public in parentcraft and healthy living.

In the new integrated service the Health Visitor is under the direction of the District Nursing Officer who delegates responsibility to a Divisional Nursing Officer.

MATERNITY SERVICE

The Area Health Authority is responsible for administering a comprehensive maternity service. Obstetrical antenatal care includes dental and medical attention. Avoidance of certain medical conditions in mothers is necessary for the health of their children. Chief amongst them are dental sepsis, nutritional anæmia, venereal disease and blood group incompatibility as between mother and child.*

Most blood group incompatibility arises in the absence of the Rh factor from the mother's blood. Statistics show that about one white mother in six lacks it—i.e. is *Rhesus-negative*. Now if a Rh-negative mother bears a Rh-positive baby (presumably with a Rh-positive father) it is probable that a conflict will arise between their blood as a result of which the mother's blood will develop antibodies which destroy the red corpuscle in the child's. The effect on the baby is to produce jaundice† and probable death either before or soon after birth. Lack of Rh-factor can be detected only by laboratory tests and one of the midwife's duties is to see that such tests are made for all her white patients. The incidence of Rh-negative blood in coloured women is very low. It does not follow that, because the Rh groups of the mother and father differ in the way described, their children will be affected. It occurs only in about 1 in 250 births and usually after one or more healthy Rh-positive children have been born.

A further reason for routine blood tests is that mothers in childbirth sometimes need blood transfusions which must be compatible with their own.

Sufficient hospital beds should be available for the care of mothers expecting complicated deliveries or first children or whose home conditions are unsuitable. Enough midwives must be provided to care for mothers in the home and ante- or post-natal clinics. The midwife works in close co-operation with the family doctor and the registered obstetrician. She must be prepared to send for the doctor when abnormality is threatened. It is her duty to notify the local area health authority (Area Medical Officer) of the birth and to notify still births, cases of jaundice, puerperal pyrexia, ophthalmia neonatorum and pemphigus neonatorum to the Divisional Nurse Officer (Community).

* In the white races Rh blood incompatibility is responsible for disease in 1 in 200 births. In 1956 0·28 per cent of primipara (a woman giving birth to her first child) and 0·35 per cent multiparæ (a woman who has had more than one child) whose blood was tested in six transfusion centres gave positive syphilitic tests.

† Icterus gravis neonotorum (Severe jaundice of the newborn).

Midwives are provided with modern equipment, including apparatus for the administration of gas and air. A maternity pack, containing all the necessary sterilised equipment, is provided free for every mother having her baby at home.

The maternity service also makes provision for sub-fertility clinics, and special arrangements are made for the care of premature infants. In many areas a " flying squad " is available for the emergency care of complicated midwifery cases, which may involve the administration of blood to the mother or baby and the resuscitation of an ill or premature baby. An ambulance service must be available for the transfer of cases to hospital.

The Maternity Nurse is one who has taken only the first examination of the Central Midwives Board. She is allowed to work under the supervision of the doctor and to nurse the mother and baby during the lying-in period. She is not allowed to undertake the whole delivery without the supervision of the doctor.

State Certified Midwives who have ceased to practise midwifery for more than a limited period must undergo a refresher course decided upon by the Central Midwives Board before being allowed to recommence practising. Practising midwives must also undergo a refresher course every five years. A midwife who disregards the rulings of the Board can be prohibited from practising.

The idea of the midwife being attached to a family medical practice has become well established and many hospitals offer facilities for family practice deliveries.

THE MIDWIFE

The midwife makes one of the most valuable contributions to the health of the community in Great Britain. As the practitioner in normal midwifery she is the person trained to help the healthy woman discharge a normal physiological function. She is trained to give skilled care and advice to the mother during pregnancy, the three stages of labour and early puerperium, and to make use of this opportunity for teaching the whole family the rudiments of healthy living.

The profession of midwifery is one of the oldest in the world, whose early history tells a gloomy story. The word " midwife " is derived from the two Anglo-Saxon words, " mede " meaning " with " and " wif " meaning " woman ", so it really means " with woman ". This describes well the role the midwife plays during labour, acting as a companion, to give encouragement and engender trust.

Before the turn of the century the birth of a baby was a family affair—the baby was born at home with the assistance of one of the members of the family or an employed untrained " maternity nurse ". Some of these people did become quite skilled, but many were notorious " Sarah Gamps". The maternity and infant mortality rates were high, and for this reason the Midwives Act 1902 provided for the proper training of midwives, and laid the foundations for the British midwifery service as we know it today. Since then, great progress has been made, and now the midwife is a highly respected member of society. From being an independent practitioner she has become an essential and important member of the health team.

From the passing of the 1902 Act great progress was made in the growth of antenatal care, and in the recognition of its value in preventing maternal and infant mortality and morbidity. As a result of this progress, helped to a large extent by the work of R. W. Ballantyne of Edinburgh, the *Maternity and Child Welfare Act of* 1919 was born. Although this was followed by a period of steady improvement as shown by more favourable statistics, it was not until 1936 that one of the greatest hazards of child bearing was minimised— *puerperal sepsis*. The greater understanding of blood compatability together with the availability of blood and the discovery of sulphonamide and later antibiotic drugs had a profound effect on the maternal death rate, and since 1936 have played an increasingly valuable part in obstetrics. Since then most mothers have chosen to go into hospital for their deliveries, and it would seem this tendency will continue. Inpatient facilities have already been increased mainly by shortening the time spent in hospital, but it is our present aim to extend them still further by increasing beds so that all mothers who choose to do so can enter hospital.

Since 1936 it has been illegal for anyone to practise midwifery in this country without being qualified to do so and registered by the Central Midwives Board. To be state certified midwives, state registered nurses or state registered children's nurses must undergo twelve months preparation, three of them in the domiciliary field. An enrolled nurse can be prepared in eighteen months, but an otherwise-untrained person must complete two years. It is now possible for students to be seconded for three months of midwifery training during their three years of general training. At the completion of the course until 1976, all trainees must have achieved success in two examinations, but an integrated one-year course with one qualifying examination has replaced the present two part training. From February 1976 all those commencing Midwifery training must undertake the integrated one-year course to qualify as a State Certified Midwife (SCM). Part-time training is also being introduced. If practice in midwifery is abandoned for any length of time after this, a refresher course must be completed to the satisfaction of the Central Midwives Board before practice can be resumed.

In Great Britain ninety-five per cent of pupil midwives are recruited from the ranks of state registered nurses, and although training and status vary from one country to another there seems a growing tendency for this to become a post certificate course.

The midwives' responsibilities towards public health can be considered under two main headings:

(1) Nursing care of mother and baby.

(2) Responsibility for health education.

(1) Nursing Care of Mother and Baby

By careful supervision and assessment during the antenatal period the midwife can do much to prevent maternal and infant mortality and morbidity, prematurity, stillbirths and neonatal deaths. Examinations during early pregnancy include blood tests for hæmoglobin and Rh factor, urine testing, weighing and examining for œdema, blood pressure reading and abdominal palpation. Such examinations enable the doctor to detect and treat toxæmia which is one of the major causes of premature labour. With our present standard of living, anæmia is not such a problem in this country, but in those where malnutrition is common anæmia from post-partum hæmorrhage is a major cause of death. During this early period the midwife is able to assess social conditions, and with the doctor, mother and husband can jointly decide on arrangements for the confinement. Mothers whose labours are likely to be complicated, including those who have had a number of children (7+) and who therefore constitute greater obstetrical risks are usually persuaded to go into hospital.

During the immediate delivery period the midwife must exercise her skill in detecting fœtal distress, so that the doctor may be called in time. She must practise a high degree of skill during labour and delivery to prevent hæmorrhage, and must be capable of resuscitating a newly born baby.

During the statutory ten days lying-in period she helps the mother to adjust herself to the new arrival, encourages breast feeding or helps with the establishment of bottle feeding, and generally supervises the care of the baby who is at this time particularly susceptible to infection and severe chilling.

(2) **As a Health Educator** the midwife has a unique opportunity, for she has contact with the whole family at a time when tension, anxiety and excitement make them receptive of counsel and advice.

Group teaching in collaboration with health visitors, physiotherapists, obstetricians and general practitioners is conducted in hospitals and health clinics. These classes give future mothers opportunities of sharing confidences, comparing experiences, and forming friendships, and enable midwives to reassure them. Much apprehension is removed from their minds as they learn about the stages of labour, the use of analgesic apparatus and the value of relaxation, so they can approach their hour of childbirth with pleasant expectation rather than with fear. Included in the classes are discussions on diet, hygiene, exercise, preparation for breast feeding, and the baby's requirements.

In all these discussions father is encouraged to take part so that he can have a better chance of understanding how his wife will be affected, and how he can best help. Together they can decide if his presence at the birth of the child would give help and support. In this way confidence can be built up in the parents and this is especially valuable with a first baby, so that both can assume parenthood with reasonable self-confidence.

When the second or third child is expected the midwife can observe the reactions of the other children and can give advice to avoid problems which might arise through jealousy. She tries when necessary to encourage an attitude of acceptance to congenital deformity, and offers advice on how to obtain the best treatment. She has an important role in giving support to special families.

Finally, the midwife plays her part in preventing mental ill health. By her skilled observation and delivery she can prevent mental subnormality due to birth injury. By her efforts to reduce stresses and strains of childbirth she may prevent mental ill health in the parents. By aiming to establish satisfactory relationships in early life she might prevent mental breakdown in later life. Indeed the midwife strives to promote mental health in every possible way.

And what of the midwife herself? To do this work effectively she must be sufficiently mature to have come to terms with herself, to have gained knowledge of the psychological and social needs of the community, and of the resources available for its help.

In the United Kingdom we are fortunate not to be burdened with overwhelming problems of illiteracy, poverty, ignorance and superstition, nor to suffer unduly from problems of malnutrition and infectious disease. Unfortunately these problems do affect many countries. The British midwife with the advantages of past experience and her present-day training has a vital part to play internationally. With her attributes of skill and sympathy, given time and opportunity, she can do much to raise the standard of public health throughout the world.

THE SCHOOL HEALTH SERVICES

Area Health Authorities are responsible for the medical and dental inspection and treatment of school children, for which the Secretary of State is required to make provision under Section 3 of the NHS Reorganisation Act 1973.

The purpose is to identify, as early as possible, any departure from normal, to ensure that appropriate advice and treatment is being obtained and to advise the local education authority, the school, the parents and the pupils of any health factors which may require special consideration during the pupil's school life.

THE HOME-HELP SERVICE

One of the provisions of the National Health Service Act was that of the Home-Help Service. From past experience it was realised that many of the community services provided such as that of health visiting, home nursing and midwifery could not work efficiently without adequate domestic help. Originally the service was organised by the Local Authority or by voluntary organisation but now the responsibility for organising the service rests with the newly appointed Director of Social Services. Suitable women are interviewed, selected and trained and a panel of helps kept available. The help is paid an hourly rate or a weekly wage by the Local Authority. The user of the service pays full cost or reduced charges according to his means. The home is visited by the organisers and the work supervised as necessary. Shopping, cooking, washing and cleaning are the duties of the home-help.

Two developments have tended to increase demands on this service. Maternity services are so arranged that mothers can be admitted to hospital for the delivery only, to return home fairly soon afterwards. The help service is flexible to meet this new demand and, where possible, the home-help goes to the home to meet mother, father and children before she is required to help. An emergency service is the second section that has developed, emergencies including, in addition to maternity cases, acute sickness, post-operative cases returning from hospital to relieve bed shortages, mental illness and special families.

To offset some of the extra demand the number of helps required for tuberculosis has decreased in recent years.

With the greatly increased expectation of life and the aftermath of two world wars, many old people are left without families to care for them. Their children go out to work or move to new housing estates. The majority are far happier and remain much more active in their own homes, but can stay there only if they have help with shopping and domestic chores. Not only are they happier and healthier but the cost to the authority is far less than it would be to maintain them in residential homes. It is the elderly who make the greatest demands on this service but it is also used effectively for households caring for the chronic sick, the disabled and for those coping with the arrival of a new baby—whether mother is at home or in hospital—and for households where the mother is ill.

This service offers to people without special qualifications an opportunity of helping their fellow citizens. Apart from practical aspects, the regular attendance of a kindly and understanding home-help can be a great comfort to a lonely old person, or to one having a worrying time through family sickness. Father can often manage to look after the children at night and in the morning, if a home-help is available throughout the day. This excellent arrangement also avoids the necessity for splitting up the family and temporarily fostering the children in other homes or nurseries.

Some authorities maintain special panels of home-helps who have volunteered to help in households where there is tuberculosis: and some provide a night sitting-up service.

In 1968 a further Act made it a duty for the local Health Authority to provide adequate home help service for people handicapped as a result of illnesses or congenital deformity. This Act also provided for the supply of laundry.

More recently a nation-wide study of the home-help service has been undertaken to find the extent to which the service complemented or eased the burden on other services, whether the service was satisfactorily organised and deployed and the extent of unmet need.

Other services which may be provided by the authority or by voluntary organisations are the supply of nursing equipment (air-rings, bed rests, commodes, cradles, etc.): a laundry service particularly for bed linen and night clothes: and a service of meals-on-wheels. This latter can ensure that old folk have a good, well-balanced and well-cooked meal two or three times a week. Where such a service is available it is highly appreciated—the kindly person who gives it can so help by giving the lonely old person another visitor to look forward to. Meals-on-wheels are available in most areas for anyone who is house-bound; recommendations for this service are made by general practitioners and the cost subsidised by the local authorities.

The aim in providing all these facilities is to ensure that medical care in the home is a practical possibility.

The Chronically Sick and Disabled Persons Act 1970 imposes a duty on Local Authorities to make arrangements for the completion of a register of all such persons and help where needed, to obtain information as to need and to publish information as to existence of services available.

RENAL DIALYSIS

It is estimated that about 7,000 people die every year in England and Wales from kidney failure. While the majority are elderly a significant number—about 2,000—are young adults 15–55 yrs and a very small number are children.

In the absence of other serious disease lives can be prolonged substantially by kidney machine treatment (renal dialysis) or by kidney transplant. Renal dialysis can be done in special centres or alternatively in the patients' own home.

In January 1968 government approval was given in the U.K. for patients' homes to be adapted to make it possible to install kidney machines for their use. The equipment is provided by the hospital and guidance is given on the provision likely to be required and on the hospital's area of responsibility.

At present only about half those suitable for treatment will have the chance of either dialysis or kidney transplant. This is largely a matter of finance; the expense is heavy; equipment and trained staff are costly; kidneys for transplant are hard to obtain, and there is a shortage of specialist facilities.

With home dialysis it is essential to teach the patient to use the equipment himself. To achieve success the home must be suitable for adaptation, and there must be a close relative or friend willing and able to give emotional and physical support. The patient must be capable of using his intelligence and self control and must want to live.

Each treatment takes eight to ten hours and must be repeated three times a week. For convenience, treatment sessions are best arranged overnight. Initially a period of six to eight weeks in a dialysis centre is necessary for the patient to learn the special skills required. It is obvious that machines are more economically used in a centre than in a patient's home.

The outlay for the equipment is in the region of £3,000 and for the initial training approximately £1,000 with a further £1,000 per annum needed for disposable and other items used. Efforts are being made to produce a much cheaper, self-sterilising machine which will cut drastically the time required for each dialysis.

Survival figures are impressive but in spite of this, because health problems and frustrations for the patient are considerable, and expense for the nation cumulative, many experts are of the opinion that kidney transplant, where appropriate, is the more attractive long-term aim.

Kidney transplant is relatively cheap. In the hands of the experienced surgeon the operation is not especially complex and necessitates a stay in hospital of only two to three weeks. Drugs are relatively inexpensive and although medical, nursing and laboratory care requires highly skilled and correspondingly highly paid staff, these are required for only a limited time. Unlike the dialysis patient, the transplant patient does not become a permanent liability on the country's finance. Efforts are being made to ensure a good supply of well matched donor kidneys and research directed toward solving the problem of rejection.

THE NATIONAL ORGAN MATCHING SERVICE

This service (NOMS) was established on 1st February 1972, at the Regional Transfusion Centre, Southmead Hospital, Bristol, in the newly established county of Avon. One of its main aims was to remove the non-medical work load connected with matching kidney and donor, from the surgical and laboratory staff involved in the surgical operation.

Previously the work involved in tissue matching for kidney transplant had had to be done by the surgeon and tissue typing laboratory staff and this had been a tedious and time consuming task.

The main aim of the service is to find the most suitable recipient for the available kidney, and then arrange the most appropriate method of transport of the kidney between the donor and the recipient hospital; these may be hundreds of miles apart or more, or may even be in different countries.

To do this, the service is equipped to centralise information; to build up a number of experienced lay staff who can locate, with the least possible delay, the best matched recipient in Europe for each donor kidney that becomes available, and then arrange the most appropriate means of transport.

The scheme has been described as " Dial a kidney ". Where a suitable kidney is available the hospital personnel dials NOMS by telephone or telex and the duty officer takes the matter on from there. It must be understood that no cadaver kidney is ever removed until brain death has been irrevocably confirmed by total cessation of heart activity, and the permission of relatives given.

To enable the duty officer to proceed with the work of organ matching a computer is stored with clinical details and the tissue typing of all patients awaiting transplant in Britain and Eire. In addition, the computer contains details of all patients throughout Europe for which there is a clinical need for priority for a kidney transplant.

Details of blood grouping and tissue typing are determined locally and the results sent to Bristol. Within moments, the computer prints out three lists for use by the duty officer, each containing details of 10 potentially suitable recipients for the kidney.

The first list are those best matched and most urgent in the immediate locality. The second list are those within four hour journey by rail, road or air, and the third list are those best matched anywhere in Britain.

Time is of paramount importance; the time lapse must not exceed 12 hours—every hour saved increases the likelihood of success. Perfusion machines are still in the experimental stage but may, if successful, extend the time interval with safety.

If no suitable recipient is available in Britain or Eire the kidney is offered—by telex—to the European network. There are three main centres for this:

1. Eurotransplant—Leyden.
2. Scandiatransplant—Aarhus.
3. France transplant—Paris.

With this link-up there is an effective pool of about 2,500 recipients.

All forms of travel are used to transport the donated kidneys in especially designed containers with the least possible delay. They may be sent overseas by scheduled, commercial or passenger air flight; by air taxi service, or by the recently formed Voluntary Air Wing of the St John Ambulance.

The journey is monitored by the NOMS duty officer who can reroute a kidney if required. The receiving unit gets about one hour's notice of time of arrival. Securicor staff may co-operate when a kidney is transported by road.

In 1973 about 500 kidney transplants were performed in the U.K. It is hoped that, as this service develops and the community becomes more understanding, an increasing number of patients will be able to benefit each year from kidney transplantation and an increasing number of healthy young adults will donate their kidneys for this purpose. Those wishing to do this should obtain a kidney transplant donor card from their family doctor.

THE PSYCHIATRIC SOCIAL WORKER

The Psychiatric Social Worker is an especially trained person who deals with the social problems of patients who need mental health care.

Much of what is said of the Medical Social Case Worker (page 243) applies to the Psychiatric Social Worker; but whereas the former is dealing with patients suffering physical illness, the latter is concerned with those suffering mental illness. Her basic training is similar, but she has specialised knowledge of mental health and illness. A psychiatric social worker is trained to be an important member of the medical team—a medical caseworker, whose aim is to help the patient help himself. Much of her work is done outside hospital, visiting patients in their own homes and visiting and advising relatives making preparation to receive someone home from a mental hospital. Anyone who has been a patient in a mental hospital needs help with rehabilitation.

The Psychiatric Social Worker is now under the direction of a County Director of Medical Social Work Service who is in turn under the general administration of the Director of Social Services. This worker is based in hospital or in the General Social Work Department.

MENTAL HEALTH

In 1954 a Royal Commission was set up to enquire into conditions in mental hospitals and hospitals for mental deficiency, and into the law relating to this branch of medicine. A full report was ready by 1959 and as a result of its recommendations a new Act was placed before Parliament.

The Mental Health Act 1959

Passed on 1st November 1960 the name of the Act was as follows:

" An Act to repeal the Lunacy and Mental Treatments Act 1890 to 1930, and the Mental Deficiency Acts 1913–1938 and to make fresh provision with respect to the treatment and care of mentally disordered persons and with respect to their property and affairs; and for purposes connected with the matter aforesaid."

Nineteen-sixty was declared Mental Health Year and marked the beginning of a new era, when mental disorder was brought into line with physical disorder. The Mental Health Service of the future will be a live and all-embracing one, with close co-operation between Regional Health Authorities and Local Authorities. It is hoped that fuller use will be made of other statutory, social and voluntary agencies.

Two main principles are emphasised.

(1) That as much treatment as possible in and out of hospital should be given to informal patients (about 95 per cent. of patients have treatment informally at present).

(2) That ample provision should be made to allow for the compulsory removal to hospital for all patients whose condition warrants it, and for their comfort when so detained.

The three main considerations must be the treatment of the patient, the liberty of the subject, and the protection of the community. The aim of the new legislation is to ensure that comparable provision is made for mental and physical illness, particularly in regard to informal admission to hospital. The standing in law of mental hospitals is now exactly the same as that of other hospitals. It is expected that psychiatric units will be set up within general hospitals—this has already been done in many centres.

Members of the medical and nursing professions can do much to help the general public to alter their attitude to mental illness, and to remove the stigma often attached to it. There is much prejudice yet to be broken down.

It is hoped that more outpatient and community care will be provided, that more combined team case discussions will be held, that " halfway " houses will continue to be set up to bridge the gap between hospitals and the outside world, and that more separate provision will be made for elderly patients suffering from senile dementia.

Every effort is already made in some cities to introduce a more realistic and satisfying element into the provision of employment for chronically mentally ill patients, and, since little of this kind of work is possible inside hospital, special outside workshops have been created.

Patients are employed as in a factory, clocking in and out, and are paid by results. Some hospital authorities act as contractors and distributors.

In 1959 the Ministry of Labour recognised such workshops as sheltered, thus enabling patients working in them to be placed on the disabled persons register.

Mentally subnormal, psychotic and neurotic patients receive help and training from government subsidised industrial rehabilitation units which cater for a variety of needs.

Another new idea was inaugurated in Bristol in 1960—a unit specifically orientated to the needs of the long-term psychiatric patient. The Industrial Therapy Organisation, known as I.T.O., is a non-profit-making company. Initially patients travelled to and from work by special bus, but now some patients live out in the community. A normal five-day week is worked by most. One of the earliest activities was a very successful car-washing service.

Following satisfactory adjustment to employment in the I.T.O. small groups of selected patients have been able to progress to work in normal factories and efforts are made to find them good lodgings. For those however who are incapable of making this double adjustment, special hostels catering for up to ten patients under the supervision of specially trained wardens are provided. Every effort is being made to extend the provision of these hostels.

Through this new and enlightened approach to their problems and with the help of present-day drugs—tranquilisers such as chlorpromazine—it is hoped that many patients will recover from the effects of long institutionalisation, and will become independent and useful members of a sympathetic community, which will learn to accept them and offer them a helping hand. One aim in the future must be to avoid such institutionalisation whenever possible.

Some terms used in the repealed Acts were considered unsuitable for everyday use, because they had become generally regarded as objectionable. With the full operation of the Mental Health Act the terms "Mental Deficiency", "Mental Defective", "Idiot", "Imbecile" and "Feeble-minded" have become obsolete, and the rigid distinctions previously drawn between mental illness on the one hand and mental deficiency on the other have been removed. "Mental Disorder" is introduced as a term covering all forms of mental ill-health, and four main categories of mentally disordered patients will be recognised as those suffering from:

(1) Mental illness.
(2) Severe subnormality.

(3) Subnormality.

(4) Psychopathic disorder.

The two groups subnormality and severe subnormality together cover the range of disorders previously included in the term Mental Deficiency.

The term "psychopathic disorder" is defined as "a persistent disorder or disability of mind (whether or not including subnormality of intelligence) which results in abnormally aggressive or seriously irresponsible conduct on the part of the patient, and requires and is susceptible to medical treatment".

Part II of the Act deals specifically with local health authorities' services. As has already been mentioned it requires Mental Health Officers to be appointed. It also permits the provision of residential and other accommodation for the education of mentally subnormal children.

Other Acts having a bearing on the same problems are the Education Act of 1944, the National Health Service Act of 1946 and The National Assistance and Children's Acts of 1948. From the Spring of 1971 the responsibility for the education of the mentally handicapped is transferred from the Department of Health and Social Services to that of Education and Science.

During the past few years the number of mentally disordered persons in care has increased.* There has been a steady expansion of services and an improvement of facilities but much more improvement is still needed. Day centres, hostel care and sheltered work shops are increasing, but, substantially increased facilities must be provided before the needs of the mentally disordered are fully met. Limitations of money and manpower hamper progress.

In England only 6 per cent of mental patients in hospital were compulsorily detained at the end of 1972. The main role of the hospital is to provide treatment and preparation for return to life in the community.

Although the number of in-patient admissions has increased, the length of stay has been much reduced and the number of beds substantially decreased—156,000 in 1953 to 121,000 in 1973. Increasing emphasis is being placed on out-patient and day-patient treatment.

At the end of 1972 there were 136 mental illness hospitals and 124 mental health departments in general hospitals.

* Over half a million people in Britain are suffering from a diagnosed mental illness. At any one time about 125,000 are in hospital.

The Mental Welfare Officer

The Mental Welfare Officer (either sex) can be described as a social worker provided for in the 1959 Mental Health Act. This Officer has replaced, in part, the " duly authorised officer ". As yet there is no specified training, but many are qualified nurses with experience in psychiatric and social work. They are employed by local authorities to carry out specific statutory duties in respect of patients requiring or receiving mental health treatment. In addition to statutory duties they may have responsibilities in connection with the care and after-care of mentally disordered children and adults, with home visiting, training centres, clubs, etc., and various others assigned to them by the authority.

In some cities this work is already well organised with mental welfare officers working with consultant psychiatrists, and attending outpatient clinics and hospital case conferences. These officers also arrange for all compulsory admissions to psychiatric hospitals or to psychiatric wards within general hospitals. They work in close co-operation with general practitioners, and a rota system is maintained so that a mental welfare officer is available by day and night.

In connection with work of social care and after-care, hospital and local health authority services have been integrated to enable social workers to give patients continuous attention through all phases of their illness. Mental Welfare Services now form part of the total Social Services provided for under the Social Services Act of 1970.

PREVENTION OF MENTAL ILL-HEALTH

The late Sir Winston Churchill said of the Mental Health Act of 1959, "This must not be a sofa, but a spring-board. . . . A spring-board for further fruitful effort by all those who are working to illuminate the dark corridors of the human mind with reason restored and hope reborn."

This is indeed a stimulating challenge, for how do we prevent mental ill-health without first knowing its source?

At present about forty-two per cent. of the National Health Service beds are occupied by mentally ill patients (this includes mentally subnormal). In addition many such patients are being cared for at home, in most cases supported to some extent by one or more community services, and many patients attending hospitals and family practitioners do so with physical symptoms caused by emotional stress and strain (anxiety neurosis).

Until we know its causes we cannot suggest any direct measures for the prevention of mental ill-health, but if stress and strain are contributory factors then indirect measures are possible and are in the hands of society. We must aim to produce a positive programme for mental health, which will promote general peace of mind, emotional balance and inner stability.

To do this we must all strive for the abolition of poverty and malnutrition, for a general increase in our standards of living, for better housing and social planning, for further development in maternity and child welfare services. Given these improvements, together with adequate education for everyone, we might be successful in raising moral standards, lessening the incidence of alcoholism, drug addiction and sexually transmitted diseases. This in turn could check the increase in incidence of broken homes, illegitimacy and crime.

Improved standards alone are not enough—they must be in step with character training, and an educational environment which teaches inner self control. It must be emphasised however that these are only *indirect* measures, which may help to minimise stress and strain.

It has been suggested (by Bowlby) that many cases of mental breakdown have their root in early childhood; lack of stability, security and affection all have their aftermaths. Voluntary services such as marriage guidance councils (see page 247) can help in this direction; much overdue rethinking of hospital practices to allow children and parents frequent and regular access to each other in all types of hospitals. Although much progress has been made in this respect there is still resistance in certain areas.

The new Suicide Act of 1961 which recognises suicide to be a sociological and psychological problem rather than a crime is another challenge. An effort on the part of all of us to prevent loneliness (see page 233) which can drive human beings to such desperate lengths, is a real need. This applies particularly to old people, many of whom deserve happier and easier lives.

Mental subnormality is a slightly different problem. There is no convincing evidence of heredity, so even if compulsory family control were possible it would not necessarily help. We do however now know that a small number of mentally subnormal children are born with biochemical disturbances (phenyl ketonuria) that may be detected and treated with encouraging results. A simple " napkin test " taken during the first three months of life by a health visitor will detect this abnormality. Recently the Phenestix testing for phenyl ketonuria has been replaced by screening by the Guthric Blood Test.

Not only will this information help to obtain effective treatment for the child, but detection of carriers and family control are important preventives. From the Spring of 1971 the responsibility for the education of the mentally handicapped is transferred from the Department of Health and Social Services to that of Education and Science.

Lastly and probably most important of all is the awakening of the public to the new idea of mental ill-health. The education of a society that will abolish the stigma attached to mental illness; a society that will accept with sympathetic tolerance and understanding the less fortunate with permanent mental handicaps or recurrent breakdowns.

We should all remember that this *is our* problem, and say to ourselves, "This might be me or my child." Together we can be effective.

LONELINESS

One of the sad things about growing old is the tendency to survive one's contemporaries, to lose one's close friends or life-long partner; but perhaps the most damaging of all is to lose one's usefulness. Unfortunately, too, there is often a gradual decline of respect and sympathetic understanding amongst younger members of the family.

During the lifetimes of our older generations there have been two world wars—many are living today who lost their husbands in the 1914 war and their sons and daughters in the 1939 war.

Another reason for this problem of our age is the scattering of families amongst the new housing estates, together with the break-up of city street communities. Loneliness among old folk can mean great unhappiness as well as mental illness and members of the various community services are trying to find means of relieving it. Old folks' social clubs etc. fill a need, but so often the most lonely and needy are too proud to admit it, and will not join in.

Day centres help to provide old people with companionship and activity, hot nourishing meals at prices they can afford. Some provide workshops and hobby clubs, advice bureaux and launderettes. Participation in the activity of these centres gives our senior citizens the opportunity to feel part of community life again.

Loneliness is however not confined to the elderly. The adolescent, the young adult and the middle aged can suffer desperate loneliness even in crowds. It is much easier to feel lonely in big cities like London, New York or Paris than it is in the country. It is possible and not unusual to feel lonely in a communal residence such as a nurses' residence or students' hostel.

Obviously loneliness often has its root in the character of the lonely one. Perhaps he lacks ability or willingness to talk or cannot share other peoples' problems and sorrows or even enjoy their pleasures. His need is none the less real however, and if someone more fortunate can find a way of breaking down his reserve he will have performed a most worthy social act. Some can do it easily: most can if they set their minds to it.

Our patients can sometimes feel lonely as also can some of our colleagues. We must remember too that sometimes the people we least expect to suffer from loneliness do so.

The physically and mentally handicapped have additional reasons for loneliness and need special help. The need to communicate their feelings to someone who cares about them is very real.

They do not want our pity—they want our positive help. This can best be given as friendship and companionship. Such facilities as provided in day centres are an obvious asset to these categories.

THE CHALLENGE OF RETIREMENT

It has been said that life should be lived to the full until death. In spite of the provision made in Britain to prevent disease and maintain positive health, it is a constant cause for concern that a large number of men and women who retire at the age of sixty to sixty five are chronically ill, while some have retired early on grounds of ill health or strain. The expectation of life for a man retiring at this age is about twelve years, for a woman it is a little longer. 20 per cent of the population of Britain are over 60, and about 13 per cent are over 65.

Every day about one thousand people reach retiring age and it is sad to reflect that many who retire suffer from sickness created by their own habits or by lack of life satisfaction. Many of the seeds of ill health are self sown: smoking, drinking, lack of exercise and over-eating are some of the contributory factors.

The senior citizen wants nothing less than to become a "drop-out". Although retired from a regular wage earning role, he still wants to be accepted as an active member of society: a member of the special group he has felt part of for most of his life, a loved parent, a wanted neighbour and a respected citizen.

A nurse, retired for some years from a senior hospital post, gives some twenty hours a week to work as a home help. She was asked if, after a lifetime of service to the community, she didn't think she deserved a rest. " That's just it," she replied, " after a lifetime of being in the community, I can't just drop out of it." In less westernised cultures this does not happen because special duties are assigned to the elderly members of the family which fulfil this need.

Retirement problems are found far more in urbanised countries, especially where family patterns, responsibilities and traditions have changed radically in the past century. When people get accustomed to comfort and amenities being within their spending power, an abrupt drop from salary to pension may require a fundamental change in their way of life. Graduated contributary pension schemes are being introduced to partially overcome this. Most retired people have to consider seriously a reduction in holidays and entertainments and, if hobbies have been expensive ones, these often have to be curtailed. The ordinary amenities previously considered essential may have to be reduced: such things as daily newspapers, periodicals, visits to the hairdresser, running a car. While these adjustments are serious enough, health need not be endangered. It is endangered, however, when pensioners find themselves in circumstances in which adequate winter heating and a fully nutritious diet are not possible because of financial embarrassment.

Boredom is an equally serious problem. For some, particularly men, it is difficult to fill the long day, whereas a woman finds it easier to busy herself around the house with domestic tasks. As the mental powers and emotional drives lessen with age, the ability to find a vital interest in a new hobby diminishes too. One suggestion is to take up one new interest extra to those previously enjoyed. If possible it is good to choose an interest that stimulates mental activity. Local Government news sheets advertising " What's on " are worth reading. Many free and reduced charges for amenities and entertainments can be exploited. Men and women need to have absorbing leisure occupations by the age of forty, which from then on can increase in importance, so that the change to a full-time interest in these pursuits can be virtually imperceptible.

The Government in Britain has recognised the problem to be overcome and has implemented schemes through voluntary bodies and local health authorities for " preparation for retirement " classes.

The citizen receives a pension toward which he has contributed during his working life and Social Security supplements this pension if needed. Elderly folk are encouraged to stay in the locality where they are known and where their friends are; to move into a smaller house during middle age while they are still able to make the necessary adjustments; to budget and think ahead with regard to clothes, car and furniture and to make proper provision for their belongings and family and to make a will.

In Britain advice can be obtained from the Pre-Retirement Association, 35, Queen Anne Street, London, W.1. This association organises retirement courses.

Much of the organisation of the care of the elderly and the services to maintain them in their own homes comes under the direction of the Director of Social Services and is the responsibility of the Secretary of State for Health and Social Services. Voluntary and statutory services combine to keep the elderly in their homes. Home nurses, health visitors and home helps spend a large part of their time on the elderly. Good neighbour and friendly visiting services are becoming more established, and other services are provided such as chiropody, sitters in, night attendants, special laundry facilities, day centres, clubs, recreational workshops and meals for old people.

The National Old People's Welfare Council heads a network of more than fifteen hundred old people's welfare committees throughout the country which provide for consultation and co-ordination at local level between statutory and voluntary services.

Under the National Assistance Act, homes for the elderly and infirm are registered. Newer ones are being established for thirty to fifty residents and nearly one thousand of these have been opened during the last twenty-five years. Many local authorities have, under the Housing Acts, provided an increasing number of smaller dwellings and flatlets for those who can be independent with help. County Councils make grants towards the cost of providing wardens and other welfare services.

While progress is being made, much more is needed. The group previously grossly neglected is that which includes psychogeriatric patients who have spent a good part of their lives in hospital but who could live in the community if suitable housing and help were available.

The challenge facing the community and the health service is tremendous: to keep all citizens really fit, fully alive, free from preventable disease until death occurs. The greatest needs are money and manpower. If the community could discipline itself to use available resources more economically, much could be done toward achieving a better deal for the elderly.

THE HEALTH CENTRE

The idea of Health Centres originated from the National Health Service Act of 1946. Local Authorities were given power to provide, equip and maintain centres where general practitioners could see their patients and make full use of local authority services; where ante and post natal clinics could be held and health visitors, home nurses and midwives could meet regularly together with doctors, to discuss their patients. Other facilities varied but most of the early centres included services such as those given by nutritionists, physiotherapists, dentists and social workers, and a few provided diagnostic and pathological services. Nursing staff were on call to deal with minor ailments and emergencies during the day and night.

Centres were situated in the area of the community they served. This gave those working in them the opportunity of becoming friendly advisors of their clients. Experienced health visitors were in charge.

The extension of this service in the first twenty years of the National Health Service was limited to a few large centres. One of the earliest was the William Budd centre in Bristol which was opened in 1952. This has proved a great asset to the local community.

At one stage the Health Services Council decided that such centres were uneconomic on the scale envisaged in 1946, but the climate of opinion changed to such an extent that by 1970 about 229 centres were functioning in England. In 1971 the Government gave local authorities top priority for capital expenditure toward this development, and as a result by the end of 1973 468 health centres were in operation in England. In addition 153 were under construction and many more planned.

About ten per cent of doctors now work in health centres—centres run by health authorities and manned by multi-disciplinary teams of doctors, dentists, nurses, midwives, health visitors, pharmacists, social workers and others, so to provide an all-round primary care service and in some cases consultant and other out-patient services.

Advantages of such health centres are numerous, but particularly they provide the means to improve the standard of general practice. The provision of modern accommodation and facilities tends to encourage consultation between doctors and enables them to specialise along their own lines. There are economic advantages in the shared use of expensive equipment, nursing and secretarial help. Also opportunities are provided for health education and the planning of preventive medicine.

Such centres can, in addition, provide for the treatment of minor ailments and recovery services. This is not only of benefit to the patient but also saves valuable hospital time and manpower. They make possible the implementation of an appointments system with economic advantage to doctor and patient. Queues are eliminated, thus reducing risk of infection and the doctor can be more prepared for his next patient if he knows who it is.

Lastly and most valuable of all is the opportunity for providing a community based health service whose clients can benefit from the full use of all the local authority social, medical and voluntary personnel.

CHIROPODY SERVICE

This paramedical therapy service is provided by the Regional Health Authority on a District basis, for the elderly, the physically handicapped and expectant mothers. The service is given in clinics, old people's homes as well as in clients' own homes. This is a valued service greatly appreciated by those who make use of it.

The chiropodist is accountable to the Medical Administrator.

THE PUBLIC HEALTH INSPECTOR

This officer, who is under the direction of the Medical Officer of Health, is concerned with administration and application of the sanitary laws. He investigates complaints of insanitary conditions; deals with verminous premises; is responsible for the inspection of food and water and of any premises used for the preparation and selling of food. He has responsibilities connected with safe milk supplies and often acts as meat inspector. He investigates reports of nuisances—water pollution, smoke or offensive trade smells; is concerned with the control of infectious disease, by helping with the investigation of the cause and the disinfection of premises. Special officers under his direction—rodent officers—are responsible for the destruction of rats and mice.

The qualifications of this inspector are prescribed by regulation. Some take Diploma courses controlled by the Public Health Inspectors Education Board and more recently some are undertaking a B.Sc. degree in Environmental Health.

THE AMBULANCE SERVICE

A free ambulance service is provided by day and night for any person mentally or physically ill who must be conveyed to or from hospital. Expectant and nursing mothers may also use this service. Patients may be conveyed by ambulance, sitting-case car, or by train. Drivers and attendants in charge of these vehicles are all fully trained in first aid.

In most areas the " 999 " telephone call system for an emergency is used. Anyone dialling this number should state clearly details of the place of the accident or illness, the name of the injured person (if known) and the nature of the illness or injury. The " 999 " call is immediately and automatically connected to a special line in ambulance control room. As soon as a call is received an ambulance is dispatched to the scene, or in some cities may be called by radio telephone while travelling in the area. It is sometimes found, in street accidents particularly, that calling for the ambulance may be delayed because everyone present thinks another person has done it.

As a result of the ever increasing severity of road accidents, particularly those that occur on motorways, some ambulances are now manned by medical and nursing crews especially trained to use life saving equipment and linked directly by radio to accident departments of hospitals. It is important for the ambulance personnel to work in close co-operation with the local police, fire and civil defence services.

Although less than ten per cent of ambulance journeys are concerned with accidents or other emergencies, they account for more than half the total cost of the service.

Non-urgent cases and those requiring to attend for out-patient treatment, or at a special clinic, may have transport provided if it is really necessary, but this must be authorised by a responsible member of the health team.

Since the beginning of this service returns show a steady increase in the number of cases carried by health authority ambulances. More purpose built ambulance stations are being planned and commissioned and ambulance crews now have more opportunity to undergo basic training courses. An Ambulance Service Advisory Committee is constituted to make recommendations.

With the establishment of the Integrated Health Service and reorganised administration, responsibility for ambulance services has now been transferred from local government to Regional Health Authority.

A Regional Ambulance Officer is appointed to advise the RHA on the organisation, development and control of ambulance services in the region. He provides this advice in consultation with the Regional Medical Officer and ensures that Area Health Authorities plan for the ambulance service in close collaboration with each other.

THE SCHOOL HEALTH SERVICE

This service has developed from the School Medical Service set up in 1907. As with the National Health Service, emphasis is placed on positive health so the service is referred to as school health, not school medical services. The Local Authority responsible for the administration of the National Health Service Act 1946 is the same as that for the Education Act 1944. In most areas, up to 1974, the Medical Officer of Health was also the Principal School Medical Officer. From April 1st 1974 medical and dental inspection and treatment of children at school is the responsibility of the reorganised N.H.S. It is considered that this is in the interest of child health generally and that the effectiveness of the service is dependant not only on links with other health services but also on its successful operation within an educational context. Confident relationship between doctors, nurses and teachers is important particularly when dealing with handicapped children.

Each Area Health Authority has a senior doctor responsible for child health including school health, also senior dental and nursing officers. Child and school health needs are under constant government review. The service aims to perform four main functions:

(1) The periodic medical inspection of school children. All children should be examined three times during their school life. The parent is invited to be present at these examinations and the school nurse, teacher and parent discuss with the doctor the state of health of the child.

(2) Minor ailment treatment and consultative advice is available for those who need it. Speech therapists and chiropodists, as well as orthopædic, eye, skin, ear, chest and heart specialists can be consulted. Many authorities have their own child guidance services.

(3) The assessment of physically and mentally handicapped children is a most important function. The local education authority will act on the advice given to provide special educational facilities and treatment.

(4) The school dental service is a specialist service and most authorities also run orthodontic clinics.

The supervision of the conditions in which school children live and work is also important. Children must have proper lighting, heating, washing and toilet facilities. The service is also concerned with preventive measures to combat infection—immunisation, vaccination, miniature X-ray examination of the chest, etc. It is also interested in the practice of physical education and the teaching of healthy living.

The health and education services hope to promote in the children physical, moral and spiritual well-being so that they will learn to make intelligent use of the health services. One cannot stress too much the part the parent has to play—the aim should be a three-cornered partnership between the school health service, the teacher and the parent. It is hoped that the time spent at school will be the beginning of a full and useful life, so that as children grow up they will develop their own lives and those of their children in the correct pattern.

School Meals

Education Authorities are responsible for providing school meals for all children attending maintained schools. The cost of labour is met from public funds. Parents who wish their children to have school meals are required to meet the cost of the raw materials, unless, subject to a means test, they are awarded free meals. The school dinner is planned to serve as the main meal of the day and should provide a substantial proportion of a child's energy requirements. It should have a value of from 650 to 1,000 calories, according to the age and sex of the child. The provision of school meals also provides an opportunity for giving social training, teaching good manners and encouraging sound dietetic habits.

Day Nurseries

Local authorities make some provision for the care in the day-time, of pre-school children (infancy to five years) in day nurseries.

This care may be necessary for the child on a long or short term basis, and is given when the parents are ill or handicapped, or existing under severe social or economic family difficulties. It is especially useful to help the "unsupported" mother who may have to work. Short term care may be needed in the event of pregnancy or sudden illness, or at other times of stress.

Day nurseries operate between 7.30 a.m. and 6.30 p.m. and the children are selected according to need. Local authorities bear responsibility for the cost and recovers part of it from the parents, who pay according to their financial assessment. As a result of the 1970 Local Authority Social Service Act, Day Nurseries come under the control of the Director of Social Services.

The nursery is staffed by trained nursery nurses under the direction of a senior registered nurse, and the nursery provides experience for training. The children are usually divided into small family groups, and where possible brothers and sisters are kept together.

There are over 300 establishments associated with the Health and Social Services approved for training nursery nurses. They are working in increasing numbers in nurseries of maternity units and in small numbers in children's wards of special hospitals, particularly ophthalmic hospitals.

Nursery accommodation is for obvious reasons more available in urban areas where indeed the need is greatest, and although this facility has been increased over recent years, it is still generally felt that the demand is greater than the supply. This is especially so on the new housing estates.

The following are connected with, but are not under the control of local health authorities.

Residential Nurseries

Since the 1948 Children Act residential nurseries have been provided by *Local Authorities* under the direct administration of a Children's Officer. Now with the 1970 legislation they come under the supervision of the Director of Social Services. As in the case of day nurseries accommodation is provided on a long or short term basis, but, although primarily they are for the pre-school child, the age range is more elastic.

Much that has been said about the day nursery is also applicable to the residential nursery which is provided when daytime care is inadequate to meet the social need of the children. It is therefore especially useful when children are dependent on one parent alone.

In some areas, family group homes are tending to replace the larger residential nurseries.

Nursery Schools

Yet another provision, this time by the *Local Education Authority*, is made for the pre-school child, the age range being clearly defined, and the service forming a part of the public education system which is free.

A nursery school is a separate establishment but children may attend a nursery class in a primary school. In either case the hours of attendance are from 9 a.m. to 3.30 p.m. during the school term only, and a mid-day meal is usually provided.

At present places in nursery schools are limited and are used especially for children of parents who must work, or for those children with a special need, but it is thought that this service will probably be extended.

In both nurseries and nursery schools every effort is made to teach the children good social habits, and to give opportunity for development through play therapy. The children are well fed, given adequate rest periods, and taught to accept a reasonable amount of discipline.

For infants and young children, nurseries and more particularly residential nurseries are not without hazards. The risk of infection is greater than in an ordinary home or foster home. Outbreaks of diarrhœa and vomiting (gastro-enteritis) are not uncommon especially during the summer months.

In addition many residential and day nurseries and nursery schools are run by private individuals and voluntary organisations, e.g. *The Church of England Children Society*—but all must register under the Nurseries and Child Minders Regulation Act of 1948.

THE MEDICAL SOCIAL WORKER

Medical social case workers are linked to both hospital and the public health services, and so for convenience will be included in this section. In recent years their true function has become more widely known and recognised. They are the social caseworkers in a medical setting—hospitals and public health field—trained to understand and handle personal and social problems directly related to illness and disease. Prior to the introduction of the National Health Service in 1948 the Almoners were not able to put their training to its fullest use because so much of their time was taken up with administrative and financial matters. Now that these duties have been delegated to others they are able to concentrate on medical social work and their contribution as members of the team is directed primarily towards the treatment and after-care of patients. Although in the main concerned with case work—helping patients to face and overcome the problems which arise from illness and, indeed, which may well underlie it and be its cause—the social worker may be involved in helping with material needs, and it is their responsibility to see that the patient knows of all the community's resources and makes the best use of them. They help the patient to help himself, and work *with* him, not for him. It is important to realise that they work on a referral basis, they are specialists offering a particular service, which can be called upon at any time the patient requires it, during *any* stage of his medical care.

In their work these social workers are looked upon as friends and advisers of the patient and, in some cases, of his relatives as well.

To fulfil this function successfully they must have a wide knowledge of all the available social services and how to obtain help from any of them. They are the people able to present to the doctor the social history and background of the patient. This information is particularly important in psychosomatic conditions, e.g. colitis, peptic ulcer, etc. They are the liaison officers between the hospital and domiciliary services provided by the family doctor and local health authorities, including health visitor, home nurse and midwife. Arranging the after-care from hospital takes much of their time; finding a suitable convalescent home, holiday, or arranging visiting for the elderly, or rehabilitation for those suffering any form of mental or physical handicap (disability); arranging assistance and training for those with special disabilities, the blind, deaf and spastic patient. It is suggested that there is a need for these social workers to be attached to group medical practises and in some regions of the United Kingdom this is being tried.

Like most other social workers, the medical social case worker has to be the sort of person who desires to help humanity, one with a sensitive and sincere understanding of people, an expert in personal relationships. Like most other professional people, she has also the responsibility of passing on her knowledge to others coming after her and to students working in other fields of social service.

For this work careful selection and special training is required. Candidates must have either the Diploma or Certificate of a University recognised by the Institute of Almoners as providing a suitable course in Social Studies, or hold a degree in Social Science which is considered a suitable academic basis for professional training. When students have completed their Social Studies course they are required to undertake a year's academic training (professional) in Medical Social Casework. This can be provided by the Institute of Medical Social Workers or taken at the Universities of Birmingham, Bristol, Cardiff, London, Newcastle or Southampton. As a result of the passing of the 1970 Local Authority Social Services Act all social work training comes under the auspices of the newly designated " Central Council for Education and Training in Social Work ".

CHILD CARE AND ADOPTION

The Children Act 1948 was based largely on recommendations made by the Curtis Report, published in 1946. Under this Act the care of healthy normal children deprived of ordinary home life was vested in the Home Secretary. Each local authority was required to discharge its functions in respect of these children through the setting up of a Children's committee and the appointment of a Children's Officer to co-ordinate and carry out the work.

Thus were born the Children's Departments throughout the country with their growing and interdependent teams of administrative staff, social workers (child care officers) and residential child-care staff.

As a result of the passing of the Local Authority Social Services Act 1970 this service amalgamated with the mental health and welfare services to form one *Department of Social Services* under the control of a *Director of Social Services*. The titles of Children's Officer and Child-care Officers are now, therefore, obsolete.

Social workers in the new service undertake a wide variety of duties entailing close liaison with field workers from other Local Authority departments and voluntary agencies, e.g. Health Visitors, Welfare Officers, School Welfare Officers, Probation Officers, N.S.P.C.C.* Officers.

These duties include investigations into complaints concerning the welfare of children; the reception of children into care and their subsequent placement and supervision; efforts at rehabilitation in the natural home where possible; duties under the Adoption Acts; supervision of children under the provisions of Child Protection Regulations (i.e. where care has been undertaken privately for reward by other than close relatives); Approved school after-care; visits to voluntary homes, etc.

The need for preventive casework has long been recognised and this has now been laid upon local authorities as a statutory duty with the passing of the Children and Young Persons Act 1963.

Children may be received into care up to the age of 17 years and may remain in care up to the age of 18 years, but a duty is laid on the Local Authority to secure the return of a child to a parent, guardian, relative or friend wherever this is consistent with the welfare of the child. There are provisions for further assistance to be given to children beyond the age of 18 years in special circumstances, e.g. for educational or training purposes. In certain circumstances parental rights over a child may become vested in the Local Authority until the age of 18 years or until appropriate legal action is taken to remove them.

Children in care are provided for in a variety of ways, but first consideration has to be given to the practicability of boarding out with foster parents. The selection of suitable foster parents according

* N.S.P.C.C. National Society for the Prevention of Cruelty to Children.

to each child's individual needs is a task requiring a high degree of skill, but the large percentage of children who do find security and happiness in foster homes is a wonderful tribute to the generosity and warmheartedness of our people. Foster parents are found in all walks of life and their selfless devotion to children who are sometimes disturbed, difficult and apparently ungrateful is too seldom recorded. More often than not they are able ultimately to forge strong and lasting bonds of mutual affection; but sometimes there is disappointment and frustration, and their only reward is the satisfaction of having extended a helping hand to a child in need.*

Children who are not placed in foster homes may be accommodated in a variety of residential establishments according to their needs. These are provided by local authorities and voluntary organisations and include reception centres (where observation, medical and psychiatric facilities are available); large and small children's homes; nurseries; hostels for adolescents; training homes; different types of boarding school. There is an emphasis in the large establishments on subdivision into smaller " family groups " each with its own substitute parent figure. The large barrack type " Home " has thus virtually passed out of existence. Small scattered "family group homes " of 8–10 children have also proved of value in an attempt to integrate the children more fully into the local community.

Voluntary organisations, many of which were pioneers in child care, continue to play a valuable part in this work. A few large and many small societies are members of the National Council of Voluntary Child Care organisations.

These small societies provide numerous homes and hostels for children and young people. They must be registered under the Childrens Act and all are subject to regular inspection.

Adoption in the United Kingdom has been legalised for the past fifty-odd years. The procedure is laid down by Act of Parliament and the Registrar General maintains a record of adopted children.†

Adoptions are arranged through the Social Services Department of the Local Authority or through private adoption societies—these must be approved and registered.

The advent of chemical contraception, the 1967 Abortion Act and the changing attitude of society toward illegitimacy, have collectively resulted in a dramatic decrease in the number of babies available for adoption.

* 1974. About 100,000 children in the care of the Local Authority.
† 1974. Towards the end of 1974 a further Children's Bill was introduced covering adoption, fostering and other aspects of children in care.

VOLUNTARY SERVICES

It might be argued that a welfare state should have no need for voluntary services, but this is not so. Voluntary organisations have been a feature of British life for centuries and to them we owe a great deal for our present pattern of social reform. We see them still playing a major role in developing citizen participation in revealing new needs, and in exposing shortcomings in the existing social and medical services. The emphasis at present must be concentrated on redistributing their resources to areas of greatest need. The present pattern envisages a productive partnership between local authority and voluntary organisations in the medical and social service fields which will encourage good neighbourliness and result in a community based service.

The National Council of Social Service and the National Institute for Social Work is examining the role and preparation of voluntary workers. The former body is working to develop co-operation between voluntary and statutory services. It provides consultant and joint action, carries out research, initiates experiments and undertakes promotional work in the United Kingdom and overseas.

Many voluntary services were, and a few are, administered entirely by unpaid officials. The majority are now staffed to some extent or are just administered by salaried officials. Those concerned with personal service or case work, employ trained social workers. Many workers give part or full time service, and an increasing number arrange training for their workers. The cost of these services is in some cases supplemented by national and local government grants.

The number of voluntary organisations runs into thousands ranging from national to small local groups. Some are religious in inspiration and all attempt to contribute toward the care and well-being of society.

The National Marriage Guidance Council is one of these organisations. The Council selects and trains men and women counsellors who offer help before and after marriage to those who seek it. There is no question of intrusion or interference. Private interviews are given to those seeking help and all counselling is undertaken in strictest confidence. Many couples are recommended by doctors and lawyers who recognise that marriage guidance counsellors have more time than they to help people find their own answers to their problems. Interviews last an hour and clients may be seen any number of times. When difficulties need professional help clients are referred to doctors, lawyers, clergy, psychologists or social workers who assist as consultants.

The Principles and Aims as rephrased in 1952 are as follows:

Principles

(1) Successful marriage, the foundation of happy family life, is ital to the well-being of society.

(2) Marriage should be entered upon as a partnership for life, with reverence and a sense of responsibility.

(3) Spiritual, emotional and physical harmony in marriage is only achieved by unselfish love and self-discipline.

(4) Children are the natural fulfilment of marriage and enrich the relationship between husband and wife; nevertheless scientific contraception, when used according to conscience within marriage, can contribute to the health and happiness of the whole family.

(5) The right basis for personal and social life is that sexual intercourse should take place only within marriage.

Aims

(6) To enlist, through a national system of selection and training, the services of men and women qualified for the work of reconciliation and education in marriage and family life.

(7) To help parents and others to give children an appreciation of family life; and to make available to young men and women before marriage such guidance as may promote right relationships in friendship, courtship, marriage and parenthood.

(8) To assist those who are about to marry to understand the nature, responsibilities and rewards of the married state.

(9) To offer counsel to those who encounter difficulties in the way of married happiness, if possible before these difficulties become serious.

(10) To work towards a state of society in which the welfare of the family shall receive primary consideration, and parenthood shall nowhere involve unreasonable social and economic disabilities.

Because of the disturbing facts which reveal that today's marriages are more vulnerable to collapse than ever before more time and energy is being devoted to education for family life itself—help in developing a good sound pattern of personal relationships with others. This educational work is a voluntary service available to schools, colleges, youth clubs and to young people in general.

The facts that should claim our serious attentions are that in the

United Kingdom one in fourteen of all marriages ends in divorce while for those who marry under twenty-one the figure is one in four. Of these girls marrying under the age of twenty, two out of every three are already pregnant. This does not account for the illegitimate children born, the number of which has almost doubled in the last six years.

The Family Planning Association

This independent and voluntary organisation should be supported by all interested in maternal and child welfare. Major religions now agree that it is wise to space ones children and plan for their arrival. It is the most obvious way of limiting the snowball effect of the world population explosion* and of enabling eventually the vast family of the world not merely to exist, but to live in freedom. Emerging and developing nations are less able to cope with this explosion than the more developed. Those more developed must face the need for more research to look into the vital requirements of the future in the form of food and space.

Family planning clinics function to give advice to those married or contemplating marriage immediately (within six weeks). Too many or too rapid pregnancies undermine health and render the mother incapable of giving the care and attention children need if they are to grow up healthy in mind and body. Wanted children bring happiness into a home, have a better chance of better food, and clothing, living conditions, education and a better general start in life.

Parents who have learnt to control their reproductive powers have a greater chance of creating a happier and more balanced home atmosphere, one more likely to have less worries, better living conditions and more time for recreation and relaxation.

Marriages planned, not forced, are truly happy occasions. Wanted children will be more likely to create successfully their own families.

By the end of 1970 all Local Authorities were providing family planning services and money is now provided to extend the services given by doctors and nurses.

By March 1976 The Family Planning Association as a voluntary organisation ceased. The work became the responsibility of the health authorities and community personnel are undertaking training courses ready to take over the work. The Joint Board of Clinical Nurse Studies is planning to supervise courses which will be run in conjunction with community staff groups at Area and Regional level.

* N.B. 140,000 more people in the world every day.

CHEMICAL CONTRACEPTION. THE PILL

Chemical forms of contraception have become established practice during the past decade, and in the United Kingdom the advent of the pill has reduced the number of illegitimate births and medical abortions performed. Forms of chemical contraception for men are also available and will probably become more widely used in the future.

Properly used chemical contraceptives are effective. Women of child bearing age are advised to seek proper advice from their family doctor or from established family planning clinics. Advice is available for single as well as married people and clients over 16 years are assured of confidentiality.

ABORTION

The Abortion Act 1967 came into force in April 1968 to legalise termination of pregnancy if two registered medical practitioners decide in good faith it is necessary. Certain criteria are listed.

1. Risk to the life of the pregnant woman.
2. Risk of injury to the physical and/or mental health of the pregnant woman or her family,
3. Risk of a child being born with serious physical or mental handicap.
4. Account may be taken of the woman's actual or reasonable forseeable environment (medico-social indications).

The operation to terminate pregnancy must be carried out in a National Health Service Hospital or in an approved establishment. The Act makes provision for staff to opt out from being involved with the operation if they object on conscientious or religious grounds.

Safeguards are given to ensure immediate treatment if necessary to save life.

The practitioner must notify every case of medical abortion but confidence is assured.

This Act does not apply to Northern Ireland.

Since 1967 there has been a steady increase in the number of notified abortions carried out in England and Wales—from 54–55,000 in 1967 to nearly 157,000 in 1972. The recent steep increase was due to women coming to England from countries overseas, particularly Europe—in 1972 just over 50,000.

In addition to NHS hospitals there were, by 1972, 55 homes

approved under the Act and 13 service approved hospitals. It is to the approved homes that most overseas women go.

It is a disturbing factor that the number of notifications of abortions under 16 years continues to increase, but this is proportional to the overall increase covering all age groups.

Abortion necessitates as a rule, a short stay in hospital; most stay in for 2–6 days. The earlier it is performed the better. It is safest if carried out before 13 weeks gestation; morbidity is doubled after this period. It is satisfying to note that the number of notified septic abortions is falling.

Various methods to procure abortion are practised; the choice is that of the consultant surgeon, and is dependent to some extent on the stage of pregnancy and age of the patient. Methods range from abdominal and vaginal hysterotomy; vacuum aspiration; paste; Laminaria Tents; combined vaginal methods and intra-uterine vaginal methods.

Several hospitals are now providing day care service for early abortions and achieve a low complication rate.

Cervical cancer

While many screening clinics for the early detection of cervical cancer are established, there is still a shortage of trained technicians and funds which together prevent further development.

The government aims to make available routine screening to all who need it and with this in view Regional Health Authorities are encouraged to provide immediate cytological facilities for gynaecologists and general practitioners. Screening is advised for all women over thirty-five at five-year intervals.

Cancer of the cervix is more likely to occur in those who have had several children and those who have lived promiscuously. Repeated damage to the cervix is thought to be a contributory factor. The number of cases notified each year remains fairly constant.

THE NATIONAL BLOOD TRANSFUSION SERVICE

Knowledge about blood has grown rapidly in the last 30 years so that blood transfusion has become an established part of the practice of Medicine. This national service began during the Second World War 1939–1945 when at the request of the Minister of Health the Medical Research Council set up four supply depots to cover London and the south-east of England. The service grew rapidly and by 1944 there were over 1,000,000 donors.*

It was during this time that citrate with glucose was developed for use as a preservative. It enables blood to be stored for twenty-one days at a temperature of $4°-6°$ Centigrade. This method of preserving blood is still used in some countries but is being replaced in many by a citrate–phosphate–dextrose solution (C.P.D.) in which blood may be stored for up to 28 days. It is known now that red cells can be preserved for many years, frozen under special conditions at very low temperature, as low as $-190°$ Centigrade. But this is not yet possible practically on a large scale.

In 1946 the National Health Service Act made provision for the existing services to be extended and continued as a responsibility of the Minister of Health and administered by the Regional Hospital Boards. In April 1974, there were 14 Regional Transfusion Centres in England and Wales and one in Northern Ireland, all of which are based in university towns; Scotland has its own service. Each service aims to serve the total needs of its region.

There are two central laboratories administered by the Medical Research Council to serve the needs of the regions. These are the Blood Group Reference Laboratory and the Blood Products Laboratory.

Each regional centre is under the control of a medical director who is employed by the Regional Health Authority. He recruits and organises voluntary donor panels, some of which are reserved as suppliers of fresh blood. Each centre is equipped and staffed for blood grouping, hepatitis testing, cross matching and the maintenance of a blood bank, and for the preparation† and distribution of sterile transfusion apparatus, blood grouping sera and blood components such as human plasma protein fraction (H.P.P.F.). The Medical Director provides a consultative service and arranges for the blood grouping and testing of ante-natal patients. Education for professional groups, lectures to nurses etc., and research are also his responsibility.

Donors are recruited with the co-operation of the Red Cross Services from people between the age of 18 and 65.‡ Young people are particularly welcomed. All donors attend sessions by appointment and provided they are in good health each gives three-quarters of a

---

* In 1969 there were 1,364,591 effective civilian donors in United Kingdom. In 1972, 1,492,000.

† Transfusion sets mostly prepared commercially and sterilised ready for use.

‡ In 1972 1,598,000 blood donotions. The number issued 1,378,000 = 3.4 bottles per hospital bed.

pint of blood. A previous history of jaundice or of certain other illnesses might make blood unacceptable. The blood collected is taken by refrigerated vans to regional centres where it is tested, grouped and banked. Each principal hospital holds a supply and occasionally supplies are available for use by general practitioners. If the blood is not used within 21–28 days the red cells are removed and the plasma is converted to H.P.P.F.

Medals are given to long service donors and although there are now large numbers of enrolled donors, more will be needed in the future if, as expected, blood is to play an ever-increasing part in saving life. It is an essential part of the United Kingdom's ordinary health service and cannot succeed without continued reinforcement by new donors.

CITIZENS' ADVICE BUREAUX

One of the voluntary services that is an adjunct to the Social Services—in that it provides a service to the community—is the Citizens' Advice Bureaux.

Most cities and towns provide this service which is independent of control and local governments and which is run largely by voluntary workers. The local government provides eighty per cent of the necessary finance.

In 1969 there were approximately four hundred and ninety Citizens' Advice Bureaux in the United Kingdom and in the region of five thousand voluntary workers.

These groups must by national policy be neutral and unselective in their services, and may not act as pressure groups.

Many open only part-time and in general at times more convenient to the worker than to the users.

PORT HEALTH SERVICES

The primary object of a health service at sea and air ports is to prevent the importation of dangerous infectious diseases or unsafe food into the country. In the unified service instituted in April 1974 local responsibility for port health comes under the control of the Community Physician, who is responsible to the Regional Health Authority. In London a single port authority covers areas of more than one authority.

Under the Commonwealth Immigrants Act 1968, any immigrant

including dependants, may be medically examined at the port of entry, and may be required as a condition of entry to report to a community physician with a view to necessary medical treatment being arranged.

Arrangements are now made for the medical examination of prospective commonwealth immigrants in their country of origin. Prior and in addition to this, examinations take place at ports of entry. A few persons are refused entry on health grounds.

New regulations also came into force in 1968 to extend the definition " ship " to include hover vehicles.

BACTERIOLOGY AND PRINCIPLES OF ASEPSIS

SOURCES AND SPREAD OF INFECTION

Sources of infection

The source of a pathogenic microbe which causes a disease in a human being is either another human being or an animal.

Most infections come from human beings, who may themselves be suffering from the disease or may be healthy *carriers*. Thus if a child develops measles the other children in the household will probably catch it, if they have not already had it. Similarly, infection may be transferred from patients suffering from tuberculosis, typhoid fever, dysentery, influenza, the common cold and so on. But sometimes a person may develop an infection, even although he has not been near an apparently infected patient. In this case, the germ has probably come from a person who is a healthy carrier. The existence of carriers complicates considerably the problem of controlling infectious diseases. It is comparatively simple to *isolate* a patient who has measles, and thus reduce the risk of his passing the virus to susceptible people, but healthy carriers cannot be distinguished without bacteriological study and hence are sometimes undetected sources of infection. A healthy person can become a carrier of pathogenic microbes following an attack of some disease, after which the germs of that disease continue to live harmlessly in his body (e.g. typhoid carriers); or it may be that the microbes are unable to cause disease in the carrier, because of his high degree of immunity, but can do so in others less immune; or the level of immunity may fluctuate in the same individual, so that a carrier may fall victim to his own germs.

Many people act as carriers of pathogenic organisms from time to time. Almost half the population, for instance, carry the staphylococcus—the cause of boils, wound sepsis and septic spots—at some time, in their nostrils. Some normal people carry pathogenic streptococci in their throats. During a poliomyelitis epidemic there are more healthy carriers than sufferers from the disease; the carriers excrete the virus in their faeces or in their saliva, and are more important agents in the spread of disease than the actual patients.

If it were not for this, we could control poliomyelitis simply by confining sufferers in isolation hospitals; but while isolation has some value, it is not in itself enough to prevent the spread of poliomyelitis in the community. The same considerations apply to many other infectious diseases, for example the common cold.

Some organisms which cause disease in humans come from animals. Thus, the bovine type of tubercle bacillus and the organism of Brucellosis may be spread to human beings in the milk of infected cows. A slightly different variety of Brucellosis transmitted in goats' milk, was first described in Malta by Bruce and was named Malta fever. Anthrax, some of the food poisoning bacteria (salmonella group) and some pathogenic viruses and protozoa also come from animals, which are the primary sources of the infections. There are many other examples of animal diseases which can afflict humans, but they are greatly outnumbered by the primarily human infections.

Transmission

The routes and vehicles of infection are many and varied, and a particular kind of microbe may be spread from person to person in several ways. Generally, the mode of spread depends to a large extent on the organs affected by the disease. Thus germs that affect the throat or lungs are likely to be coughed out and to float in the air, and to be inhaled by a new victim; whereas the germs which cause diarrhœa and typhoid fever are spread chiefly in the faeces of the patient or carrier, which contaminate the food or drink of the new victim.

There are four main modes of spreading pathogenic microbes:

(1) **Alimentary**—the faecal to oral route.
(2) **Contact**—direct or indirect; and inoculation
(3) **Airborne Spread**—via contaminated dust or droplet nuclei.
(4) **Certain Insects.**

(1) *The Alimentary Route* is of particular importance when the intestinal canal is the site of the disease and the pathogen is excreted in the fæces of the patient or carrier who acts as the source of the infection. This is the main way in which the germs of typhoid fever, paratyphoid, dysentery, cholera and salmonella food-poisoning, reach the victim. But certain other diseases, not primarily intestinal, can also be spread by the alimentary route, notably poliomyelitis and infectious hepatitis.

How do microbes travel from the excreta of one person to the mouth of another? They may be conveyed on hands, toys, babies' feeding bottles, etc. or they may be swallowed in contaminated water or food. In the past, water contaminated by human sewage was responsible for many outbreaks of typhoid fever, paratyphoid fever and cholera (see Section 2). Water-borne outbreaks have become rare, following the improvement in water supply. They are still common in countries with primitive sanitation and water supplies.

Milk and milk products such as ice cream can convey the microbes of intestinal disease if a dairy worker is excreting the microbes or if contaminated water is used to rinse the churns. (Milk may also convey bacteria from infected cattle, as we have seen.) These risks are minimised by cleanliness of dairies and healthy cattle, and by heating the milk in *pasteurisation*.

Many other foodstuffs may become contaminated by microbes of gastro-intestinal disease, either by being handled by persons who are themselves excreting the germs or by flies that have crawled on excreta. And some foodstuffs of animal origin may be contaminated by organisms originating from the animal itself. Bacteria of the salmonella group, common causes of food poisoning, in fact are primarily pathogens of animals and birds. Thus, an outbreak of food poisoning may be caused by meat coming from an infected animal, from which organisms may be spread, in the slaughterhouse, factory or kitchen, to other food products; it may be caused by infected eggs (especially duck eggs); or it may arise through human contamination of food. Food may also be contaminated by rats and mice, which often excrete salmonellas.

The prevention of infection spread by food consists partly of measures to ensure that only healthy animals are used, e.g. by food-inspection and by regulation of slaughter houses and food factories; and partly of measures to avoid contamination during preparation of food for the table. It is important that food-handlers go off duty if they suffer from diarrhœa or vomiting, and remain off until pronounced fit to return; and—most important—that *all* be strict in their personal habits. Hands should always be washed thoroughly with soap and water, and dried with *individual* towels after visits to the lavatory, and before handling food; and good washing facilities should be provided. The staphylococcus of septic fingers also may cause food poisoning, although they are not of intestinal origin. People with septic fingers should not handle food.

If, in spite of precautions, pathogenic bacteria do contaminate foodstuffs, the outcome depends largely on the number and virulence of the microbes. It may be possible to swallow a few pathogens without suffering harm, whereas to swallow a large number of the same germs would result in an attack of diarrhœa and vomiting or of some more serious disease.

Some articles of food, particularly made-up meat dishes, rissoles, gravy, cold chicken, also cream and the like, are very good culture media for bacteria. Such foodstuffs should be stored for as short a time as practicable, and should be kept cold, so that pathogens, even if present, cannot multiply. *Adequate refrigerated space is an important protection against food-born diseases.* Frozen poultry should be thoroughly thawed before being cooked.

(2) *Contact.*—Direct contact with a diseased tissue may result in infection. This is the principal mode of transmission of infections caused by delicate organisms that die quickly outside the body—e.g. the venereal diseases, syphylis and gonorrhoea. But germs are more often transferred from an intermediary object which has previously become contaminated. This is *indirect contact.* The object is called a *fomes* (plural, fomites).

Indirect contact is an important mode of spread of the bacteria of boils and septic wounds. Many other diseases such as smallpox, chickenpox and intestinal and respiratory infections may also be spread by indirect contact. Indeed the number of diseases which can be transferred in this way is very great. The actual articles on which the germs may be stored are many and various; a child's toy, the thermometer used for more than one patient, crockery, hand towels, baths, blankets and—very important—the hands of doctors and nurses. Fomites are legion.

Soil and road dust may contain spore forming bacteria from animal manure, e.g. gas gangrene and tetanus bacilli.

Microbes may be inoculated into the tissues by contaminated syringes and needles and injected fluids.

(3) *Airborne Spread.*—When a person sneezes and coughs, and to a smaller extent, when he speaks, he sprays out fine droplets of saliva and other secretions, often invisible but containing germs from the mouth and respiratory passages. The smaller droplets quickly dry up and their residue, containing microbes, consist of tiny " droplet nuclei " which may float in the air for long periods and be inhaled by other people. Thus airborne spread is of particular importance in the spread of pathogens which affect the respiratory tract, to cause sore throats, colds, diphtheria, and whooping cough, tuberculosis and many other diseases. Air may also be contaminated by small particles of microbe-laden dust from bedclothes, garments, handkerchiefs, and from the skin. Squamous cells, conveying bacteria

from the skin are constantly being shed from the surface of the normal body. Some of these bacteria may be pathogenic, e.g. staphylococci. Airborne bacteria may cause wound infection in operating theatres.

The risk of spread of airborne disease is very great in a crowded room or badly ventilated cinema or hospital ward. The risks may be reduced by avoiding overcrowding, by correct use of clean hand-kerchiefs and by adequate ventilation.

(4) *Certain Insects* can spread microbial diseases. Sometimes the insect acts as a " mechanical " agent, e.g. the fly, which feeds first on fæces and then on food in the kitchen transfers microbes on its feet.

More often, however, the insect carriers of disease transfer the germs by sucking blood from a human being or animal suffering from the disease and then biting another individual. In this way, certain mosquitoes transfer the protozoa of *malaria* and the virus of *yellow fever*; fleas transfer the *plague* bacillus from rats to human beings; body lice transfer the organisms of *typhus fever* from person to person.

These are a few examples of the many known instances of transfer of germs by insects. Clearly, insect borne disease can be prevented by eliminating the insects. The reduction in flies, by the removal of their breeding grounds; the destruction of mosquitoes, by draining ponds and swamps where they breed and by means of insecticides; the reduction of the louse population, by personal cleanliness and good laundry facilities, have all played a large part in the control of preventable disease.

TISSUE CHANGES IN RESPONSE TO INFECTION

When micro-organisms invade body tissues certain changes take place. Suppose for example that staphylococci enter the tissues around the nail bed. The body will respond by increasing the blood supply to the part—the increased blood will cause the typical signs of inflammation—redness, swelling, heat, pain and loss of function. The cause of redness is obvious; swelling and heat are produced by the excess blood entering the part and not being able to escape at an equivalent rate; pain is caused because of tension, the tiny vessels are all distended and nerve endings are pressed upon. In the nail bed pain is often described as being " exquisite " because of the generous distribution of sensitive nerve endings in that region, and because tension is increased by the hardness of the nail. Because of the tenderness, the body will resist any movement and the part tends to cease functioning in the ordinary way. The local reaction of the tissues is defensive. As a result of these changes, described as hyperæmia with exudation, the fluid part of the body (the plasma) oozes out through the minute vessel walls taking with it polymorphonuclear leucocytes, which are capable of amœboid movement. These white cells immediately move into the attack and fight the invading organisms by ingesting them (phagocytosis). The presence of opsonins (see page 264) and the vitality of these fighting cells determines to some extent the result. If they are entirely successful in destroying all the micro-organisms and clearing them away, then all signs of inflammation will subside and we describe the result as one of resolution—the inflammation has resolved itself.

This process of resolution is obviously most favourable and desirable, but is often not possible. The battle between the phagocytes and the organisms may have been a fierce one, with casualties heavy on both sides, and some surrounding tissue cells must have been destroyed. This debris forms thick white or yellow fluid called pus. Staphylococci, streptococci and other organisms which cause pus to form are known as pyogenic (pus-forming) bacteria. A collection of pus surrounded by tissue is called an abscess. If left alone the battle continues in this localised area, and if the body defences win, one of two things happens: the pus becomes gradually absorbed by the blood cells, or, more often, finds its way through the path of least resistance and breaks through to discharge on to the surface of the body or burst into the nearest cavity. A sample of this pus under the microscope makes an interesting and informative picture. Dead blood and tissue cells, with micro-organisms, will be seen together with white cells in the process of performing phagocytosis. All this activity following exudation is called localisation and suppuration.

Now suppose that during any of the three stages just described the organisms win the battle. They get past the local defences and enter the lymph vessels and small blood vessels. Fortunately for us, at strategic points along the lymph vessels are placed lymph nodes (also called lymph glands). A lymph node is a small structure which contains large numbers of white cells called lymphocytes. The fluid in the lymph vessels is called lymph. Any bacteria in it are usually filtered out in the nodes. The node may then become inflamed (*lymphadenitis*) with increased blood supply and swelling, and polymorphonuclear leucocytes enter it to destroy the bacteria. Thus a person with a septic finger may develop tender swellings in front of the elbow or under the arm due to lymphadenitis. If the lymph vessels themselves become inflamed, red streaks may be seen under the skin where they pass up the arm (lymphangitis). Suppuration (pus formation) may occur in the lymph gland. But if the bacteria have been prevented from passing, the body is still protected from serious harm.

Now suppose that the invading organisms are so virulent and numerous that the glands are quite unable to stop them, the result will be serious because the organisms will stream in large numbers through the lymph glands and enter the blood stream where the lymph channel enters a vein, and so becomes quickly transported to all parts of the body. If the bacteræmia is sustained for sufficiently long, by more and more organisms spilling into the blood stream, the antibacterial defences of the blood, itself normally so powerful, may be overwhelmed and the bacteria may be actually multiplying in the blood stream. This serious condition is called *septicæmia*. The patient is very ill, and if untreated is likely to die in a few days. Multiple abscesses may develop in various tissues; this condition is known as *pyæmia*, an old fashioned term signifying "pus in the blood".

During the early stages of this infection, the patient is probably aware only of the pain, swelling and other effects of local inflammation. However the bacteria produce chemical poisons, called toxins, which soon diffuse into the blood capillaries, and are carried round the body, and are responsible for a feeling of illness (malaise). If the infection remains localised, probably nothing more than slight pyrexia, headache, anorexia, furred tongue and a general feeling of lethargy will result, but if it is severe, the patient may be really feverish and toxic, exhibiting all signs and symptoms of an acute toxæmia, i.e. high temperature, increased pulse and respiration rate, severe headache, rigor, anorexia, nausea and vomiting, constipation or diarrhœa. Children may have convulsions, and both children and adults may become delirious. In addition to causing such general symptoms, common to many infections, the toxins of certain bacteria have specific effects on particular tissues. Thus a throat infection by hæmolytic streptococci may damage the glomeruli of the kidneys, or the lining of the heart in a small proportion of people, especially children, with resulting acute nephritis or rheumatic endocarditis. The toxin of the diphtheria bacillus damages heart muscle and certain nerves, and so a patient with diphtheria may develop acute heart failure or paralysis of various muscles. Tetanus toxin damages the central nervous system.

Two other results are possible. A state of *cold war* may exist between the invading organisms and the tissue cells; neither can succeed completely and so there is continuing evidence of inflammation. This is a most undesirable state of affairs. The organisms continually damage the tissues both locally and in other parts of the body, so the body's defences are kept active and its resources drained. This is referred to as *chronic infection*. It is undesirable for many reasons: chronic infection once established is hard to eliminate, it produces a gradual change in the tissue structure which leads to interference with function. Chronic infection is a strain on the body's resources of energy, resulting in a general lowering of vitality and resistance to other infections.

Another result of inflammation due to infection is death or necrosis of the tissue. If on a small scale, it is referred to as a slough—for example the core of a boil—if on a large scale the word *gangrene* is used. This in itself and on a small scale is not serious, but can become a danger. Dead tissue lying dormant in the body is a potential source of trouble and a good breeding ground for micro-organisms. Necrosis and gangrene are by no means always due to infection; they may also be caused by restriction of arterial blood supply to a tissue.

A useful indication of active infection in the body is the number of white cells circulating in the blood stream. The body reacts to infection by many sorts of bacteria with increased activity of white cell precursors in the bone marrow, which produce increased numbers of polymorphonuclear leucocytes (polymorphs) to circulate in the blood stream. The result often is an increase of white cells from the normal value of about 5,000–10,000 per *cmm*, up to 20,000 per *cmm* or even more. This is known as *leucocytosis*. Generally the more acute the infection, and the more tissues involved in it, the higher the leucocytosis. Leucocytosis is a feature of infection by many organisms, especially the pus forming cocci, but by no means all. Tubercle bacilli, salmonella bacilli, and viruses are examples of important pathogens which often have little effect on the white cell count. Another indication of infection is body temperature. In the absence of infection there is a constant balance maintained between heat production and heat loss. This results in normal temperature, which averages 37°C. When infection is present the activity of the body is increased and the temperature raised. In the very severe and acute infections it is greatly increased.

This increase in temperature is a defence reaction, since pathogenic microbes usually die more quickly at high temperature than at normal body temperature. The temperature is raised by increased muscle activity—sometimes with shivering and rigor. If the patient is left untreated the body temperature will often alternate between high and normal or subnormal, and the typical swinging temperature chart results. Sometimes the rise of temperature is so great (hyperpyrexia) that vital organs might be damaged, and it is then necessary to cool the patient by tepid sponging or in other ways.

Before efficient antibacterial drugs became available (antibiotics and sulphonamides), the bacteria-killing effect of high temperature was sometimes used in treatment. Thus, high temperatures were deliberately produced by infecting patients with malaria (afterwards cured by quinine) in the treatment of late results of syphilis.

Toxins. Many pathogenic bacteria produce toxins, but do most of their damage by actually invading the tissues. Some important pathogens, however, have very little invasive power, but make up for this lack by producing exceedingly powerful exotoxins. (See p. 195.) The best example is the tetanus bacillus, which, if it enters a wound (especially a dirty, deep wound where dead tissue excludes oxygen supply) may multiply and produce its toxin which diffuses along the nerve fibres to the central nervous system which it damages, causing the convulsions of tetanus. Another important toxin producer is the diphtheria bacillus. It causes a type of sore throat which in itself is not serious, but the diphtheria toxins produced by the bacilli in the throat lesion enter the blood stream and are carried round the body to cause serious damage to the heart and to peripheral nerves.

RESISTANCE OF THE BODY TO MICROBIAL DISEASE—IMMUNITY

As we have seen, pathogenic microbes may be transferred to healthy people from time to time. Good hygiene can often prevent this transfer, but some microbes are bound to get past the barriers. Fortunately however this does not always result in disease; for the pathogen has yet to overcome a formidable obstacle, the resistance in immunity of the host.

As one would imagine, the more virulent the pathogens the fewer are required to cause disease. Thus, as we have seen, disease may often be prevented by means which reduce the numbers of bacteria, even if their actual presence cannot always be avoided. Hence the importance of careful handling of food, the use of a refrigerator in the kitchen, good ventilation, etc. Immunity may be *innate* (*inborn*) or *acquired*.

Natural Immunity can be due to several normal defences. For reasons we do not understand it tends to vary in different species, races, families, and from time to time in an individual. The skin and mucous membranes, if healthy and intact, prevent the entry of bacteria into the underlying tissues. The importance of the part played by these coverings is shown by the prevalence of skin infections and of infections which often follow chemical and mechanical damage to the mucous membranes of the air passages, e.g. bronchitis and broncho-pneumonia following inhalation of irritating fumes or " smog ". Several of the body fluids, blood, mucus, saliva, tears, vaginal secretion, and so on, contain chemical substances which damage bacteria. Hydrochloric acid in the stomach kills many bacteria swallowed in food.

The white cells in the blood, called *phagocytes*, are mainly polymorphonuclear cells, so called because of their peculiar many-shaped nuclei. They can move like amœbæ, and by virtue of this amœboid movement are able to crawl between the lining cells of the blood capillaries, leave the blood and enter the actual tissues. The phagocytes do this when stimulated by the presence of invading bacteria in the tissues, and having reached the invaders they ingest them and destroy them. Many phagocytes may themselves be killed in the process, but are readily replaced by the proliferation of their parent cells in the bone marrow. Phagocytes are essential for the day-to-day defence of the body. This is well demonstrated by what happens when, owing to a diseased condition, phagocytes are not produced. In this disease (agranulocytosis), the patient suffers from very severe infections, chiefly of the mouth, throat and other mucous membranes, which may eventually cause death.

The natural immunity of the individual presents a formidable and complex defence system to the would-be invaders. Good health and a good diet are said to increase an individual's resistance to infection. But there are very many infections which are as readily " caught " by the healthy as by the weak (common colds, influenza, mumps, chicken-pox, are a few of the many examples which come to mind). It is probable that good general health protects an individual against the serious effects of an infection, even if it does not prevent him from catching it. Thus, measles is more serious in a weak infant than in a healthy one.

Diabetes mellitus is a good example of a non-infectious disease which lowers the resistance of the body to infection. Staphylococcal infection of hair follicles (boils) may be more severe in diabetics than in other people. Lack of vitamin A from the diet leads to an unhealthy state of the mucous membranes of the eye and throat, with consequent susceptibility to infection. But susceptibility to infection does not increase if the patient takes an ordinarily well balanced diet. This contains all the essential vitamins and there is no need to supplement it.

In addition to the natural immunity which we possess from birth, immunity to a variety of infections may be *acquired*.

Acquired immunity may be the result of natural or artificial causes, and may be actively or passively acquired. Active immunity to a particular microbe or its toxin may be acquired naturally, by surviving an attack of the disease (e.g. measles). Sometimes the attack which confers immunity may have been so mild that the person was unaware of it. Thus, when diphtheria was commoner than nowadays, some people became immune as the result of a subclinical infection. An active immunity against a disease may also be acquired artificially, by injecting a killed or " attenuated " suspension of the causative organisms, or an altered toxin (toxoid),into the patient. This method was introduced in 1796 by Jenner, a doctor who practised in Berkeley, near Bristol. He immunised people against smallpox by inoculating them with living cowpox virus. The cowpox virus is closely related to smallpox virus, and causes a trivial infection in man, which, however, is followed by immunity to smallpox.

The bacteria that inhabit the normal skin, mouth, alimentary tract and vagina also play a part in resistance to disease. Their presence helps to prevent invasion by other microbes. Anything that damages the normal flora may result in infection by pathogens. Thus, the administration of large doses of antibiotics sometimes leads to inflammation of mouth and bowel, due to the elimination of normal flora and multiplication of other organisms.

Vaccinia is the Latin name for cowpox, and from it came the words *vaccine* and *vaccination*. Nowadays, vaccine means a suspension of any organism which is injected in order to stimulate active immunity. Other living but attenuated vaccines which are thus used nowadays are those against yellow fever, B.C.G. vaccine against tuberculosis, and the Sabin type of poliomyelitis vaccine. The organisms in the vaccines have been attenuated, i.e. modified to make them harmless without killing them. Sometimes it is unsafe to use living vaccines, and killed or inactivated vaccines are used instead, e.g. T.A.B. vaccine, used to stimulate immunity to the enteric fevers (typhoid and paratyphoid A and B). In the case of a disease caused by an exotoxin produced by the pathogen it may be better to immunise against the exotoxin, rather than against the microbe itself. Thus, active immunity to diphtheria and tetanus is produced by injecting, not the exotoxin (which would be much too dangerous), but attenuated derivatives of the exotoxin, known as diphtheria toxoid and tetanus toxoid. As a result of active immunisation with diphtheria toxoid, the death rate from diphtheria was reduced to 0·12 per million in 1954 compared with over 200 per million at the turn of the century.

Active immunity to a microbe or its toxin, whether artificially or naturally acquired, is the result of a reaction of the individual's own body. Proteins from the microbes, or their toxins, act as *antigens*. (An antigen is a foreign protein, i.e. foreign to a person's body.) The introduction of an antigen into the body stimulates the body to become immune. This immunity is *specific*, i.e. operates only against similar microbes or toxins. Sometimes the immunity is due to changes in the tissue cells themselves and is known as *cellular* or *cell-mediated* immunity; and sometimes it is due to *antibodies* produced by special cells (lymphocytes) in the body. Antibodies, like antigens, are proteins. They pass into the person's blood and tissues and combine chemically with the corresponding antigen if it is present there. If the antigen is a bacterial toxin, the combination with antibody neutralises it. Such an antibody is known as antitoxin. If the antigen is a part of the microbe itself, it may be damaged or made more susceptible to attack by phagocytic white cells. Antibodies which do this are called *opsonins*; they are, as it were, the sauces that make microbes palatable to phagocytes.

In some diseases active immunity is mainly cell-mediated (e.g. tuberculosis, typhoid fever, many virus infections); in others it is mainly due to antibodies (e.g. diphtheria, scarlet fever). In many, perhaps most microbial diseases, however, active immunity is partly due to antibodies and partly cell-mediated. Active immunity usually lasts for a long time, sometimes even for life. The body, having once responded to a particular antigen, as it were " remembers " how to respond and quickly produces antibody or the necessary cellular changes again if the need arises. This is why people rarely suffer from a second attack of measles, a disease due to a single *antigenic type* of virus. But it is common experience that some infectious diseases can attack the same person repeatedly. The explanation usually is that the microbes of such diseases exist not as one type (as in measles) but as several different antigenic types. That is, these microbes differ from one another in some of their antigens though they all have the same effect on the person's body. Thus most people catch many colds and have several attacks of influenza during their lifetime because, unlike measles, there are many different types of common cold virus and of influenza virus.

There is another kind of acquired immunity—*passive immunity*. In this, the individual becomes immune through the presence in his blood stream of antibody manufactured by *another* individual. Natural passive immunity in an infant may result from the diffusion, across the placenta, of antibody present in the mother's blood before the infant is born. Thus, newborn infants are usually immune to measles for six months, because their mothers have usually had it and still carry the neutralising antibody in their blood stream, from which it diffuses into the fœtal blood stream. In the past it was believed that, as in some animals, colostrum and breast milk supplies this antibody, but is now known that this does not happen in humans. Passive immunity is conferred artificially by injecting antibiotics that were manufactured by other individuals. Thus, a child may be given passive immunity to measles by injecting pooled concentrated antibiotics (knwon as gammaglobulins), made from the blood serum of several human adults. Passive immunity to diphtheria and tetanus is conferred by the serum of horses, previously immunized against the toxins of these organisms. Serum which is used to confer passive immunity is known as *Antiserum* (or *Antitoxin* if it contains antibody against a toxin).

Passive immunity can be conferred almost instantaneously, as for example, when tetanus antitoxin is used to protect recently wounded patients against the risk of tetanus. Within a few minutes of injection of antiserum, the antibody is circulating in the patient's blood stream, and is thus available to protect the patient against the corresponding microbe or toxin. Passive immunisation is also used to treat established infections. By giving antitoxin to early cases of diphtheria, much of the toxin is neutralised before it gets to the tissues, and is therefore prevented from doing harm. But once toxin has become fixed in the tissues, it cannot be neutralised by antibody. Thus, in tetanus, by the time symptoms appear, the toxin is already in the spinal cord, and antitoxin cannot neutralise its effect, though it can prevent more toxin from being absorbed.

The main disadvantage of passive immunisation is that it does not last long. In a few weeks, the injected antibody disappears from the patient's blood stream. Thus, passive immunisation is used to produce immediate, but temporary protection. If lasting immunity is required, active immunisation must be used.

The above account of immunisation procedures may suggest the question: " Why is not immunisation used for many more diseases? "

If it is successful in preventing diphtheria, tetanus, smallpox and yellow fever, why is it not used to prevent pneumonia, influenza, the common cold, and other infections to which we may succumb? There is no simple answer. With some diseases the causative bacteria do not readily stimulate the body to produce antibodies, or the antibodies, even if present in the patient's blood, may fail to damage the microbes; or a disease, such as the common cold, may be caused by any one of many different types of the microbe; or, again, the process of immunisation may itself be dangerous. This is the case sometimes with passive immunisation. The injection into a patient's body of a foreign protein, such as a serum derived from an animal, occasionally provokes a severe reaction, known as *anaphylactic shock*. This reaction is most frequently seen in people who have previously had an injection of the same kind of serum, or in people who are subject to hay fever or asthma, but it may occur in anyone. The reaction is sometimes very severe, with collapse and faintness, and is occasionally fatal. Hence, following an injection of antiserum, the doctor keeps the patient under observation for some time, and is prepared to treat anaphylactic shock with adrenaline and other drugs. Special care should be exercised in the case of persons thought to be liable to anaphylaxis, e.g. hay fever and asthma sufferers, and persons who previously have had similar injections.

In summary, the forms of Immunity are

(a) INBORN. Due to general (non-specific) factors: intact, healthy skin and mucous membranes, leucocyte action, etc.

(a) ACQUIRED (specific)

(i) ACTIVE—*Natural*, following an attack of the disease. Due to antibody production or cell-mediated immunity, or both.

Artificial, induced by injection of vaccine or toxoid which stimulates cell-mediated immunity or the formation of antibody.

(ii) PASSIVE—*Natural*, by transfer of antibody from mother to foetus, across the placenta.

Artificial, by injection of ready-made antibodies in the blood-serum of other human beings or animals.

PREVENTION OF INFECTION

Cross Infection in Hospital. This term, in its widest sense, refers to any infection contracted by a patient who is already in hospital. The term includes non-specific as well as specific infections, whether or not they are notifiable. During the past thirty to forty years the situation has changed very much. When the so-called isolation hospital came into being, special risks were created by having in the same building groups of people suffering from different infections. At first, each ward was allocated for the nursing of one type of disease; techniques were used to prevent the transfer of infection from one person to another and great care was taken with terminal disinfection (see page 279). A very high standard was achieved in this type of nursing, and it was unusual for " cross infection " to occur, i.e. for a patient admitted to hospital with one specific infection such as diphtheria to contract another, such as scarlet fever. Although this obvious type of cross infection occurred only rarely, it has more recently been shown that much cross infection of a less obvious type did and still does occur in general hospitals. It occurs particularly with pathogenic organisms that are often carried by normal people, e.g. staphylococci, B pyocyaneus etc. and with similar organisms in wound and other infections of surgical patients. Gastro-enteritis in infants is another example of an infection that is readily transferred from patient to patient. Recognition of these problems has brought about changes in the care of patients.

The first change was mainly in mode of segregation, each patient being nursed in a separate cubicle containing all his own belongings. To a large extent this practice was successful and is still used, but it has disadvantages. The nursing of patients in separate cubicles requires a large staff, and is not very good for children. They are often lonely and unhappy and feel the separation from their homes and parents very much when they are alone. The tendency nowadays is for the doctor to encourage parents to nurse children with infectious diseases at home, if necessary with the help of the social and health services. It should be only when home conditions are unsuitable that children are admitted to hospital with infectious disease.

" Bed isolation " or *barrier nursing* also grew from the original isolation hospital, and considerable success has been achieved in nursing patients with some infections in general wards, or patients with different infections in one ward. Provided that proper and sufficient facilities are available, and that doctors and nurses interpret intelligently their knowledge of how the diseases are spread, barrier nursing may be a safe method of nursing some of the less easily transmitted diseases. Methods of disinfection should be reliable, bed spacing and ventilation good, the arrangements for disposal of linen adequate, and the health of the attending doctors and nurses carefully supervised—they should not be overworked. Overwork may not only

270 MODERN TEXTBOOK OF PERSONAL AND COMMUNAL HEALTH

lower personal resistance to disease but may also cause lowering of standards of work and thus be responsible for cross-infection.

The isolation hospital of today is very different in function from that of fifty years ago. Many diseases, then common, have become rare (e.g. typhoid fever and diphtheria). Nowadays, isolation hospitals are occupied largely by patients with tuberculosis, gastro-enteritis, dysentery, measles, etc., which are more easily and safely nursed there than in general wards. However, it is possible that large general hospitals of the future will have their own isolation wards, for the care of patients who are sources of dangerous infection.

In general hospitals, where cross infection is now a greater problem than in isolation hospitals, much research in methods of prevention has been carried out since the Second World War.

It has been shown that hands, bedding and clothing are often responsible for transferring pathogens from person to person, by indirect contact. Some organisms may live and even multiply in weak disinfectant solutions, saline lotions etc. Airborne transmission of organisms has been found important in operating theatres where wounds have to be exposed for long periods; but even in the theatre, contact infection is often a greater risk. Some bacteria, notably anti-biotic-resistant staphylococci, have become established in hospitals by " colonising " the noses and skin of doctors and nurses and patients noses, wounds and other skin lesions. Infected wounds and lesions are usually more dangerous sources than noses since they contain more organisms. By no means all persons colonised by staphylococci will suffer harm, but some develop wound sepsis and other infections.

The discovery of methods of typing staphylococci was a valuable result of research. By distinguishing between different strains of the organism it often enables sources of outbreaks of infection to be identified.

Methods to prevent this type of cross infection are many and varied, and require the conscientious co-operation of everyone—doctors, nurses and domestics. A high standard of cleanliness in the patient, his belongings, and his surroundings must be maintained. Aseptic methods, such as non-touch dressing techniques, must be performed carefully and intelligently. However, since despite good general standards of nursing care cross infection may still occur further measures are necessary. These will depend on the circumstances, the nature of the infecting organism, the type of patient involved and so on. Generally speaking, control measures will consist of:

(1) Elimination of *sources* of infection (i.e. persons with open lesions and sometimes carriers). This may best be achieved by isolation or barrier nursing, and by occlusive dressings. Best of all, it may be possible to prevent more patients from becoming sources. Thus, in maternity nurseries, the use of a disinfecting dusting powder on the babies' skins and cord stumps will often protect them against colonisation by staphylococci, and thus prevent them from becoming sources.

(2) Routes of transmission by indirect contact should be eliminated or reduced.

Hands and Towels

a) Roller to be replaced by individual ones or mechanical hand driers. The hands need great care. As elsewhere on the body, the skin harbours many germs. Some are deep in the glands of the skin and cannot be removed. Others, on the surface, picked up by touching contaminated objects, can be removed by thoroughly washing and drying the hands. Wet, dripping hands easily transmit infection. Disinfectant soaps are an additional precaution for use in operating theatres but generally not needed in wards. Brushes should not be used, except occasionally for nails which should be kept short. Brushing the skin roughens it. The hands should never be needlessly contaminated nor allowed to touch a wound.

b) *Bedding:* to be disinfected frequently: mattresses and pillows to be enclosed in waterproof covers: blankets to be disinfected after each patient's use.

Because this is difficult with woollen blankets, cellular cotton ones which can be boiled, are coming into more general use.

c) Baths, utensils, crockery, barber's equipment, etc., to be disinfected frequently. Properly designed shower baths are safer than bath tubs.

d) Common use articles: bath wraps, dressing and toilet mackintoshes, shoulder capes, chest blankets, occasional blankets, children's toys to be either eliminated or frequently disinfected. These articles should not be passed from one patient to another.

e) Care with disinfectants, lotions and ointments, especially those that may become contaminated with bacteria (see page 193).

f) Closed drainage of wounds, and of the bladder after operation.

g) Bedpans should be disinfected, also urine bottles from patients with infections of the bladder.

(3) Reduction of *airborne infection*. Avoidance of overcrowding, efficient ventilation, the use of a good method of bed-making—one which avoids unnecessary flapping of blankets—will reduce airborne cross infection. Other measures to eliminate dust include the use of damp or oiled dusters, and of vacuum sweepers. The modern type of flooring which can be damp mopped each day, and the use of separate dressing stations are all obvious advantages. Special ventilation systems are often installed in operating theatres. Much can also be done by simple measures, e.g. avoiding unnecessary movement and the presence of unnecessary visitors in operating theatres.

Opinions of the value of face masks vary. Properly used, they reduce the transfer of infection by droplets and hence are of value in circumstances in which droplet-spread diseases are important. But the wearing of masks by ward nurses while dressing wounds has little value as a precaution and may give rise to a false sense of security. Most bacteria in the air of wards are dust-borne, not droplet-borne, and will not be reduced by wearing masks. It is obviously important to refrain from speaking while performing a dressing, at least from speaking directly over the wound.

Where masks are used, they should be worn correctly, and not handled or lowered and raised again. To do so will contaminate the hands. A misused mask is dangerous.

Patients should be taught to cough with care and to spit into a proper receptacle. Paper handkerchiefs should be used.

It is important that all members of the hospital staff, domestic workers and porters included, should have an elementary knowledge of the meaning of cross infection, of the risks involved and of measures to prevent it. Further measures of control concern administration and hospital design, and are beyond the scope of this book.

PRINCIPLES AND APPLICATION OF ASEPSIS AND ANTISEPSIS

The word "asepsis" means complete freedom from microorganisms. An antiseptic inhibits the growth and activity of microorganisms but does not necessarily kill them all. Joseph Lister introduced antiseptics into surgery, and from his work has grown the practice of asepsis which permits use only of sterile materials.

In all dressing and theatre technique every effort is made to work in surroundings and with equipment that are completely germ-free. The area of operation, whether on the surface or inside the body, is rendered as clean as possible without damaging the tissues to be disturbed.

Knowing the requirements and habits of pathogenic micro-organisms, we now aim to provide conditions which will not encourage their growth spread. In brief, when preparing for surgical procedure, whether an operation or a dressing, it is the nurse's responsibility to see that all the instruments, bowls, towels, dressings, etc., are rendered completely germ-free by sterilisation. It is also her responsibility to see that the place to be used is clean and fresh. The nurse also has the responsibility of preparing the operation area. The patient's hair can be a potential source of infection, so the parts involved should be shaved. Creases, crevices and folds of skin need attention. Since germs are likely to survive in damaged tissue gentleness is one of the keywords of good surgery. Hæmostasis, that is the control of blood, is essential. Blood oozing into a wound area can easily produce a haematoma and become infected. Once haemostasis is complete a firm dry dressing is placed over the area and held in position by some suitable lightweight non-irritating adhesive or bandage. Provided there has been complete asepsis, and the edges of the tissue are held firmly in apposition by clips or stitches, initial healing should occur within twenty-four hours. In a well-stitched wound, infection cannot normally get in from outside after twenty-four hours. Surface dressing after this time is no longer really necessary. Nurses would do well to remember three precepts that students of surgery are taught:

(1) Absolute asepsis.

(2) Gentleness.

(3) Hæmostasis.

When surgery of any kind is practised the hands play a most important part and should be cared for as previously described. Manual dexterity is essential in manipulating forceps and handling dressings in a way that is described as a " *non-touch technique* ". With careful practice it is possible to carry out a most difficult dressing, and even insert a catheter, without touching anything that comes into direct contact with the tissues. This should be the aim of every nurse. In theatre work the surgeon must use his hands, so sterile rubber gloves are used to cover them.

Instruments used for any surgical procedure should always be treated with respect, scrubbed clean with a brush kept especially for that purpose and sterilised as required. When not in use, instruments should be kept in a special cupboard and not used for purposes other than surgery.

Where aseptic technique is practised anything that may introduce germs should be avoided as far as possible. General traffic should not be allowed through theatres, people entering should be made to cover or change their shoes beforehand. Because the nose and throat often harbours germs, it is usual to cover them with an effective mask. This face mask should be taken straight from the sterile envelope or pack and not repeatedly pulled down and replaced during operations.

In modern operations there is little antiseptic surgery. We now know that it is better to use dry sterile dressings than the wet antiseptic dressings that Lister used. However, for some purposes, antiseptics and disinfectants are valuable if used correctly and not allowed to irritate the tissues.

PRINCIPLES AND PRACTICE OF DISINFECTION AND STERILISATION

Disinfection is the process of killing microbes. Different processes of disinfection vary in their ability to destroy different types of microbe. Some microbes, particularly those with spores, are much more resistant than others.

If the process of disinfection is able to kill *all* microbes, it is called sterilisation—in other words sterilisation is disinfection powerful enough to guarantee sterility.

There are two methods of disinfection and sterilisation: physical and chemical.

(1) **Physical.** Heat is the easiest and most effective method for objects which are not themselves destroyed by heat. Heat may be moist or dry; of the two, moist heat is the most effective, bacteria being less susceptible to heat when they are dry.

(i) *Moist Heat.*—All non-sporing microbes are killed by hot water at well below boiling point. For instance, water at a temperature of 70°C kills non-sporing pathogenic germs in about 10 minutes. Milk can be freed from most bacteria, including pathogens like the tubercle bacillus, by keeping it at 66°C. for thirty minutes. This process is called Pasteurisation (although it was not introduced by Pasteur). Merely bringing water or milk to the boil will kill non-sporing organisms. In practice, boiling for five minutes is a good, safe method of disinfecting instruments (syringes, forceps, etc.) which are free from contamination by material which might contain pathogenic sporing organisms. Some people recommend boiling for twenty minutes in the belief that it will kill more spores than boiling for five minutes, but no boiling procedure can be relied upon to kill all spores.

Spores vary greatly in heat resistance. Many are killed by five to ten minutes' boiling. Some, including pathogens like tetanus bacillus, may withstand prolonged boiling. Therefore water, or steam, at a temperature higher than boiling point is used. This higher temperature is achieved in an autoclave (the principle of which is the same as a pressure cooker).

The Autoclave.—Steam is commonly used at a pressure of fifteen to twenty pounds per square inch *above* atmospheric pressure. At this pressure the temperature is 120°–126°C. and it will certainly kill all spores in a few minutes. Autoclaving is the method commonly used for dressings and other fabrics (surgical towels, etc.), gloves, fluids and solutions in sealed containers, and instruments. The actual temperature and duration used in practice vary with different materials.

The main practical difficulty in autoclaving is in ensuring that the steam penetrates the fabrics. To allow this, the air which they contain must *first* be removed usually by some form of evacuating pump. Only when all the air is out does the real sterilisation process commence. The same evacuating device is used at the end of the process to dry the goods.

Although a few minutes in steam at autoclave temperature will kill spores, in practice a longer period is allowed to make certain the penetration is complete. Thus packages of dressings are usually autoclaved at 126°C. for twenty to thirty minutes *after* the air has been removed. Higher temperatures for shorter periods are often used nowadays, especially for instruments.

(ii) *Dry Heat.*—Being less effective than moist heat, a higher temperature and longer time of exposure are required. The minimum safe conditions are 160°C. for one hour.

For the hot-air method special ovens are used. The method is good for glass and metal instruments and oily substances like petroleum jelly that are not damaged by heat; but it is unsatisfactory for fabrics (dressings, etc.) and rubber, because they are charred or destroyed at the temperature of the oven.

Hot air is best for the sterilising of all glass syringes. Nowadays however they have been largely replaced by plastic syringes, wrapped and supplied sterile by the manufacturers and discarded after use.

Burning is obviously the ideal way of disposing of infected material of little or no value. In the home the domestic fire can be used. In hospital, special furnaces are used to destroy dressings, etc.

Other Physical Agents. *Light.*—Sunlight has a good disinfecting action, although it will not destroy all microbes. The value of adequate window space and good lighting has already been stressed (p. 154).

Ultra-violet light can be used for disinfecting the surface of some objects that cannot be heated. It has little penetrating power.

Nuclear Radiation (Gamma-irradiation) is an effective sterilising agent and is used for the commercial sterilisation of dressings, catheters, etc.

(2) **Chemical Agents.** These are called antiseptics, disinfectants or germicides. The term antiseptic is sometimes used for weaker substances that can be applied without harm to skin and tissues. Very few chemicals can be relied upon to sterilise by killing all organisms.

Antiseptics are used to reduce bacterial growth in solutions and foods that cannot be kept in sealed containers after sterilisation to prevent bacterial growth, e.g. Merthiolate in solution for injection from multidose containers; benzoic acid in certain foodstuffs.

In general, no chemical method of sterilisation is as good as heat, but chemical methods must be used for disinfecting contents that would be damaged by heat. Disinfectants act by chemical action on the protoplasm of the microbe. Some in common use are as follows:

(i) *Chlorhexidine and Hexachlorophane.* Chlorhexidine (Hibitane) is useful, and relatively non-irritant for tissues. It does not however, destroy spores or tubercle bacilli. It may be used in an aqueous solution, or dissolved in 90 per cent. alcohol. In the latter form it is a good skin disinfectant. In a cream it is a useful disinfectant for the hands.

Hexachlorophane (sometimes spelt Hexachlorophene) is another chemical with a weak but persistant action. It is effective against staphylococci and streptococci, but not some other organisms. It is used in disinfectant hand washing preparations, and incorporated in a dusting powder for preventing staphylococci colonisation of the skin of infants.

(ii) Alcohols. Methylated spirit and surgical spirit are moderately powerful, but will not kill all microbes. They are often used to disinfect the skin when iodine would be irritant. They are best used diluted with water to make a 70 per cent. solution.

(iii) One group of detergents, the "Quaternary ammonia compounds", kill some forms of bacteria but are ineffective against others. They are useful in cleaning "dirty" wounds because they are cleansing but non-irritant. Cetrimide ("Cetavlon") is an example. Other detergents do not disinfect.

(iv) Halogen Compounds. Chlorine, used in compound, such as hypochlorite solutions and chloramine, are used for disinfecting water supplies, swimming baths and crockery. Chlorine is active against many viruses. Iodine is a good skin disinfectant best used in an alcoholic solution.

(v) Aniline Dyes. Flavine, crystal violet (gentian violet) and brilliant green are useful but mild germicides, for use in dermatology. They are not suitable for pre-operative disinfection of the skin.

(vi) Oxidising agents such as ozone and hydrogen peroxide destroy some bacteria.

(vii) Coal Tar Derivatives.

Black and white fluids (e.g. Jeyes' fluid and Izal) are cheap, crude coal tar preparations used for disinfecting excreta and secretions that may contain pathogenic microbes. The material should be covered by the fluid and left for one hour before being discharged down the sluice. Strong phenol or carbolic acid is a corrosive poison which will kill microbes quickly, but will also damage tissues. If diluted to 5 per cent. (1 in 20) it is effective in approximately twenty minutes. Phenol is reasonably cheap but is inclined to irritate the skin.

Cresol preparations (e.g. Lysol) when diluted to 5 per cent solutions (1 in 20) makes a soapy solution which will kill most microbes in approximately twenty minutes. Strong lysol and carbolic are dangerous caustics and should be diluted in the dispensary before being sent for use in the wards and theatres. Even when dilute, however, these substances are irritating. Much of the irritation is due to impurities in Lysol. Newer preparations of cresols, e.g. "Hycolin", "Sudol", "Stericol", etc., are safer than lysol, and as effective.

Chloroxylenol (e.g. Roxenol, Dettol) is a popular disinfectant. It is non-irritating and pleasant to use, but relatively ineffective against some bacteria such as B pyocyaneus.

(viii) Metallic Salts. Salts of Mercury (Perchloride and Biniodide) have been used in the past. Because they are poisonous and poor disinfectants they are going out of use.

(ix) Gaseous disinfectants. Formaldehyde gas is a powerful (but irritating) disinfectant in the presence of moisture. Its value is limited by the fact that it lacks penetrating power. Ethylene oxide gas is another powerful disinfectant. To be effective it must be used in special apparatus and at correct levels of humidity. Pure etheylene oxide is explosive, but this danger is avoided by mixing it with an inert gas.

Disinfection of the Skin. Disinfection of the skin can never be complete, because many bacteria are hidden in the ducts of skin glands. However, thorough washing with soap and water will remove many superficial organisms (brushes should not be used on the skin, only on the nails). The bacterial population of the skin may be further reduced by washing with a liquid soap containing 2 per cent. hexachlorophane, or by means of a chlorhexidine (Hibitane) hand cream.

Disinfection of patients' skin prior to operation is best achieved after the skin has been shaved and washed, by means of alcoholic solutions of iodine or chlorhexidine. For disinfecting skin for injections the same agents may be used. (It is often sufficient to use 70 per cent. alcohol.)

Acids and alkalis. The natural acid secretions of the body play an important part in keeping the skin and mucous membranes healthy and free from infection.

Other methods of destroying or inhibiting the growth of micro-organisms.

(1) *Soap and Water.* Thorough washing with clean warm water and soap will remove the majority of organisms, and often is all that is necessary.

(2) *The Natural Elements.*—Fresh air, the wind and especially the sun, are all effective in destroying microbes. Thorough airing of all articles and premises after use in any infectious disease is advocated.

(2) *Filtration.*—It is possible to sterilise certain liquids by passing them through special filters, but only bacteria and not viruses are held back.

(4) *Drying.* Many microbes die if deprived of moisture. Others, however, may survive. Heat is often used in conjunction with drying, e.g. sterilised dried milk can be stored for an indefinite period in a sealed container. It must be remembered, however, that some organisms will survive drying. This particularly applies to spores, although while they are dry their activity is limited.

(5) *Cold.*—Intense cold does not necessarily destroy microbes, it merely inhibits their activity.

A deodorant is neither a germicide nor an antiseptic. It is a substance which masks the smell from bacterial growth or decomposition. It does this by superimposing its own smell on that of the offending one, or by temporarily paralysing the sense of smell. Some disinfectants may have a sufficiently strong smell to act as a deodorant, e.g. phenol.

Current Disinfection is the term used to describe the process used to kill microbes in the discharges, excreta and on the belongings of any person being nursed with an infectious disease.

Terminal Disinfection describes the process whereby the patient, his belongings, his immediate surroundings and his nurse are rendered as free as possible from infection. This is done when the patient has been declared by his doctor free from infection. In the home it is usually supervised by a public health inspector. Sometimes the room is sealed and fumigated with formaldehyde and clothing and bedding are steam sterilised. This type of thorough disinfection, used for diseases of a serious nature, e.g. enteric fever and smallpox is rarely required nowadays. In cases of less serious disease, thorough airing and cleansing with hot water and soap are sufficient for the disinfection of the room and furniture.

In conclusion, methods of disinfection are probably one of the most controversial subjects, but certain facts are agreed upon:

(1) Heat is the only reliable steriliser and the best disinfecting agent and should be used whenever possible.

(2) At other times chemical disinfectants must be used—selected to suit the particular germs that have to be destroyed and the material which is harbouring them.

INDEX

Boils, 255, 258, 264
Bones, 46
Boredom, 235
Botulism, 118
Botulus botulinus, 118
Breathalizer test, 96
Bronchitis, 196
Broncho-pneumonia, 196
Brucellosis, 256
Bugs, 83

Calcium, 46
Calories, 43, 53
  definition, 43–44
Cancer, 197
  cervical, 251
Candles, 156
Carbohydrates, 42, 44, 45
Carbon dioxide, 140, 141, 144
Carbon monoxide, 142
Cardiac disease, 207
Cardiac infarction, 197
Carriers of infection, 255
Carry-cot design hazard, 125
Cellulose, 52
Central Health Services Council, 17, 28
Central Services Agency, 40
Central Services Council, 39
Cervical cancer, 251
Cess-pools, 178
  emptying, 189
Cestodes, 78
Character, 72
Chemical closets, 177
Chemical contraception, 250
Chicken-pox, 197
Child care, 214, 244–46
Child health services, 212–13
Child Protection Regulations, 245
Child welfare, 16
Children, 42, 46, 239–43
  mentally handicapped, 240
  physically handicapped, 240
  see also Battered baby syndrome
Children Act 1948, 8, 230, 242, 244, 246
Children and Young Persons Act 1963,
  90, 245
Children's Departments, 245
Children's Officer, 242, 245
Chiropody service, 238
Chloride, 47
Chlorination of water supply, 169
Chlorine, 277
Chlorhexidine, 276
Chloroxylenol, 277
Cholera, 171, 190, 257
Chronic infection, 262
Chronically Sick and Disabled Persons
  Act 1970, 224
Cimex lectularius, 83
Citizen's Advice Bureaux, 253
Citrate–phosphate–dextrose solution
  (C.P.D.), 252

Clean Air Act 1956, 142
Clean Food Campaign, 107
Cleanliness, 62–72, 136–37, 270
  food premises, 106
Clematis, 136
Clostridium botulinum, 118
Clostridium welchii, 118
Clothing
  choice of, 72–74
  choice of colours, 73–74
  choice of materials, 73
  design of, 74
Coal tar derivatives, 277
Cobalt, 48
Cocci, 192
Cockroaches, 132
Combustion products, 141–44
Comedo, 70
Comedo remover, 71
Common Services Agency, 38
Commonwealth Immigrants Act 1968,
  253
Community, 33
Community Health Councils, 20, 22–23
Community health services, 213
Community Physician, 13
Community services, 13
Composting, 175
Conduction, 148
Conservancy system, 176
Constipation, 68
Contagious disease, 199
Convection, 147, 149
Convection currents, 145
Corns, 64
Creeping plants, 136
Cresol, 277
Crickets, 132
Cross infection, 269, 270
Cross ventilation, 147
Culture medium, 193
Curtis Report, 244
Cuts, 64
Cyanocobalamine, 51
Cystitis, 196

Daddy-long-legs, 133
Dandruff, 66
Dangerous Drugs Acts, 99
Day centres, 233
Day nurseries, 241–42
Daylight, 154
Death rate, 125–26
Death watch beetle, 134
Deficiency diseases, 48, 122, 207
Degenerative diseases, 197
Dementia, 50
Dental decay, 67, 157
  see also Teeth
Deodorants, 70, 279
Department of the Environment, 30
Department of Health and Social
  Security, 17, 28, 35

Fresh air, 144
Frost bite, 65
Fruits, 51
Fungi, 193

Gammaglobulins, 267
Gangrene, 262
Garchy system, 175
Gas fires, 151
Gas lighting, 156
Gastric disturbances, 171
Gastro-enteritis, 117, 120, 243, 269
Gastro-intestinal disease, 257
Gastro-intestinal infections, 190
General practitioner services, 13–17
Germicides, 276
Glycogen, 45
Gonococcal vaginitis, 85
Gonorrhoea, 85, 89
Group therapy, 37, 105
Guthric Blood Test, 232

Habit formation, 41, 60–61
  see also Alcohol; Drugs
Haemostasis, 273
Hair, care of, 65
Halogen compounds, 277
Heaf multiple puncture tuberculin test, 203
Health care, 19
Health Care Planning Teams, 16, 20–22
Health centres, 16, 236–38
Health clinics, 16
Health education, 37, 100, 104–5, 216, 221
Health Education Council, 37
Health education officer, 105
Health Education Service, 35–37
Health Services Commissioner, 23
Health teaching, 200
Health visitor, 213–16
  training, 214
Heat transmission, 148
Heating, 148–54
  background, 153
  central, 154
  methods, 149
  open fires, 149–51
  requirements, 127
  separate units, 149–54
  temperature requirements, 153, 154
Heredity, 1
Heterosexuality, 84
Hexachlorophane, 276
Home, function and care of, 130–31
Home-help service, 6, 13, 222–24
Home nurse, 210–12
  training, 211–12
Homosexuality, 84
Hormones, 45, 53
Hospitals
  disclaimed, 13
  isolation, 269, 270

mental, 227, 228
  private accommodation, 12
Hospital services, 10–13, 15
Hospital statistics, 14
Housing, 121–26
  care of the home, 130–31
  cleanliness, 136–37
  dampness, 128
  disrepair, 128
  hazards, 124–25
  heating requirements, 127
  improvement grants, 128
  legislation, 121, 123, 128–30
  lodging houses, 129
  minimum requirements, 126–28
  movable dwellings, 129
  overcrowding, 128–30
  recommended standards, 126–27
  see also Heating; Lighting; Ventilation
Housing Acts, 121, 128
Human plasma protein fraction (H.P. P.F.), 252, 253
Humidity, 138–40
Hydrophobia. See Rabies
Hygiene, science of, 3
Hygrometer, 139
Hyperaemia, 260
Hyperpyrexia, 263
Hypothermia, 102–3
  babies, 102
  elderly persons, 102–3

Ice, disease transmitted by, 173
Immigrants, 253–54
Immunisation, 199, 203–5
Immunity, 197, 199, 263–68
  acquired, 265
  active, 266
  cellular or cell-mediated, 266
  forms of, 268
  natural, 264
  passive, 267
  specific, 266
Incineration, 174
Incubation, 198
Indian rat flea, 83
Industrial revolution, 121
Industrial Therapy Organisation, 229
Infection, 70, 129, 190–209
  airborne, 258, 272
  alimentary route, 256
  animal sources, 256
  bacterial, 117
  carriers of, 255
  chronic, 262
  cross, 269, 270
  direct contact, 258
  elimination of sources of, 271
  human sources, 255
  indications of, 262
  indirect contact, 258, 271
  insect carriers, 259
  modes of spreading, 256